*f*P

Also by Todd Tucker

Notre Dame vs. the Klan
Notre Dame Game Day

THE GREAT STARVATION EXPERIMENT

◄⟨o⟩►

The Heroic Men Who Starved So That Millions Could Live

Todd Tucker

FREE PRESS

New York   London   Toronto   Sydney

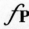

FREE PRESS
A Division of Simon & Schuster, Inc.
1230 Avenue of the Americas
New York, NY 10020

For information about special discounts for bulk purchases,
please contact Simon & Schuster Special Sales at 1-800-456-6798
or business@simonandschuster.com.

Book design by Ellen R. Sasahara

Manufactured in the United States of America

1   3   5   7   9   10   8   6   4   2

Library of Congress Cataloging-in-Publication Data
is available

ISBN-13:   978-0-7432-7030-4
ISBN-10:   0-7432-7030-4

For Susie, my inspiration

Is not this the fast that I have chosen? to loose the bands of wickedness, to undo the heavy burdens, and to let the oppressed go free, and that ye break every yoke?

—Isaiah 58:6

THE TEST SUBJECTS

William Anderson	Nashville, Tennessee	Methodist
Harold Blickenstaff	Chicago, Illinois	Brethren
Wendell Burrous	Peru, Indiana	Brethren
Edward Cowles	Port Ludlow, Washington	None
George Ebeling	Moylan, Pennsylvania	Presbyterian
Carlyle Frederick	Nappanee, Indiana	Brethren
Jasper Garner	Okeechobee, Florida	Brethren
Lester Glick	Sugar Creek, Ohio	Mennonite
James Graham	Madison, Wisconsin	Friends
Earl Heckman	Rocky Ford, Colorado	Brethren
Roscoe Hinkle	Hershey, Pennsylvania	Brethren
Max Kampelman	New York, New York	Jewish
Sam Legg	Brandon, Vermont	Episcopalian
Philip Liljengren	Chicago, Illinois	EMC
Howard Lutz	Landsdowne, Pennsylvania	Friends
Robert McCullagh	Monrovia, California	Methodist
William McReynolds	Salem, Oregon	None
Dan Miller	LaVerne, California	Brethren
L. Wesley Miller	Enid, Oklahoma	Methodist
Richard Mundy	Bloomington, Indiana	Baptist
Daniel Peacock	Richmond, Indiana	Friends
James Plaugher	Fresno, California	Baptist
Woodrow Rainwater	Fort Worth, Texas	Methodist
Donald Sanders	Sherrill, New York	CC
Cedric Scholberg (Henry)	Bingham Lake, Minnesota	Methodist

The Test Subjects

Charles Smith	Merchantville, New Jersey	Baptist
William Stanton	Woodbury, New Jersey	Friends
Raymond Summers	E. Dearborn, Michigan	Brethren
Marshall Sutton	Clintondale, New York	Friends
Kenneth Tuttle	Cleveland, Ohio	Baptist
Robert Villwock	Toledo, Ohio	E&R
William Wallace	San Anselmo, California	Presbyterian
Franklin Watkins	Pittsburgh, Pennsylvania	Presbyterian
W. Earl Weygandt	Clarksville, Michigan	DOC
Robert Willoughby	Harrisburg, Pennsylvania	Brethren
Gerald Wilsnack	Malverne, New York	Presbyterian

(Hometowns from *The Biology of Human Starvation*, p. xxxi. Denominations are those given at time of induction into the CPS, as recorded in the *Directory of Civilian Public Service*. EMC = Evangelical Mission Covenant. CC = Congregational Christian. E&R = Evangelical & Reformed. DOC = Disciples of Christ)

CONTENTS

———◆◇◆———

THE GREAT
STARVATION
EXPERIMENT

—◇—

STARVED INTO SUBMISSION

T HE SMALL TIMER on the stove buzzed and the light-hearted conversation around the table stopped. With practiced efficiency, Subject Number 20 stood, stepped away from the table, and silently walked outside. His "buddy"—a designated supervisor required to accompany him outside the lab at all times—had taken him to their friends' house in Minneapolis several times over the course of the experiment. It was the home of two elderly ladies who had somehow come to befriend the corps of test subjects. While he couldn't eat their food, just getting out of the lab and talking to people unconnected to the experiment was invigorating. At least it had been at first.

During these furloughs, Number 20 had gotten into the habit of chopping wood in the backyard until the meal was done, the dishes were put away, and the temptation to cheat and steal a morsel of food had passed. And there had been cheaters. The lapses were all too easily detected when a volunteer's weight loss suddenly veered from the predictive curve carefully drawn by Dr. Ancel Keys. Those incidents led to immediate dismissal from the experiment, stern talks from the doctor, and the implementation of new layers of supervision. Everyone knew who they were, the cheaters, the men not tough enough to finish the experiment. Number 20 had seen the shame in their eyes; he had joined in the pitying glances and the whispered reproaches. He refused to become one of them. But he still chopped wood during dinner. He knew the limits of his willpower.

In the early days, as the food was served inside without him, he would chop giant stacks of timber in the moonlight—sweating, chopping, congratulating himself on the strength of his character with each fall of the ax. Now, after months of starvation, his efforts were a farce, a charade of a strong young man helping out two widows with their chores. Either old lady could probably have picked him up and carried him across the yard. Number 20 wondered if he had strength enough to swing the ax a single time. Besides the general weakness that accompanied his malnourishment, he had also mangled a finger on his left hand the week before. It throbbed painfully. He watched the moonlight reflect on the ax's shiny blade as he walked to the woodpile.

The experiment was in the rehabilitation phase—the hard part was supposed to be over. Yet even with the starvation phase complete, the scientists controlled every bite of food in his diet, as they had for the past nine months. The volunteers who remained had been divided into four recovery groups, and each group was given incrementally more food than they had been allowed during the starvation phase. As luck would have it, Subject No. 20 suspected he was in the lowest group and, thus, given only 400 more calories a day than he had been allowed during starvation. The difference was almost imperceptible. It was a crushing disappointment after nine months of counting the hours to "R1," the day he thought he would be allowed to eat again.

The difference for his group amounted to about two slices of tasteless soy bread a day, in addition to the smattering of turnips and cabbage they were now accustomed to. He wasn't even gaining weight; in fact, he was still losing weight—which, the doctors explained, was actually his body recovering from starvation: the fluid retention caused by edema was going away faster than he could regain healthy tissue. That reasoning did nothing to cheer him up as he continued to think about food to the exclusion of all else. On good nights, he dreamt of feasts, giant steaming tables piled high with ham, potatoes, bread, and pie. On bad nights he startled himself awake with horrifying nightmares of cannibalism, wiping his mouth to see if it was dripping with blood. As he caught his breath in the gray darkness of the barracks, he would listen to the groans and the raspy, shallow snores of his friends who were suffering through tortured dreams of their own. The prospect of another three months in the lab was unbearable.

He split a log cleanly, and watched the two halves fall dumbly apart. Just that one swing of the ax exhausted him; he paused to catch his breath. He heard with sharp clarity his friends laughing inside, heard their forks scraping their plates—the scientists had confirmed a piece of folklore that said hearing improved with starvation. Was it dessert, Number 20 wondered, a freshly baked pie or a scoop of ice cream? Or were they still lingering over pot roast and gravy? He imagined slicing through the tender meat with a silver knife, feeling the blade cut cleanly until it scraped the china, soaking up gravy with a slice of warm bread, washing it all down with cold milk.

He could quit at any time, of course—several men had. He was supposed to be stronger than that, a leader of the group. He was supposed to be suffering for his pacifist beliefs, while at the same time benefiting mankind in the study of starvation and rehabilitation. Men were dying overseas in the war. Friends of his were in the fight. Hitler had starved millions. How would Number 20 be able to say that he had been not only unwilling to serve alongside the troops, but also too weak to even complete a science experiment? He knew that for the rest of his life, people were going to ask him what he did during the war. The starvation experiment was his opportunity to give an honorable answer to that question. How could he quit?

So he had stuck with it, feeling colder, fainter, thinner, and hungrier each day. When he caught a bad cold, Number 20 found himself hoping it would get worse. For days he searched his tired body for symptoms of tuberculosis . . . to no avail. He had begun to think of the hospital, with its starchy meals, as his deliverance, an honorable alternative to quitting or expulsion.

Just a week before, Number 20 dropped his car on his hand. He had jacked up his old Packard in the stadium parking lot, pretended to do some maintenance, and then pulled the pin on the jack as he set his left hand on the ground. He flinched, pulled his hand out at the last instant. He had only crushed a finger, and not badly enough to be removed from the study. The doctors were suspicious, of course, and would have yanked him from the experiment in a second if they had thought him suicidal or psychotic. He insisted convincingly that it was an accident. They took him to the hospital, but continued to bring him carefully measured meals from the laboratory's kitchen. He loathed himself for losing his nerve, and wondered if he would get another chance to fake a believable accident.

Subject No. 20 knelt on the ground of their friends' yard and stood up one of the logs he was to split. It had a smooth, flat surface, as smooth and level as a small table. He splayed the fingers of his left hand across the flat top of the log and looked at them. Like everything else on his body, they looked alien to him now. His knuckles bulged on spidery, thin fingers. His pale skin was blue in the moonlight. One blackened fingernail reminded him of his last pathetic attempt. With his right hand, Number 20 raised the ax into the air. He had to grip the handle about halfway up to put the blade in range. He barely had the strength to hold the ax, and wondered seriously if he could bring it down with enough power to do any damage. He thought about three more months of hunger, three more months of scientists prodding his body and psychologists probing his mind, with Dr. Keys watching somberly in the background, making notes on his clipboard, raising an occasional eyebrow at the graphs of the psychological inventory.

Number 20 pulled the ax down with a grunt and what remained of his strength. The blade came down straight and true. Before he passed out, Subject No. 20 watched with satisfaction as three of his fingers rolled off the log and into the neatly mown grass.

CHAPTER ONE

HIGH ALTITUDE STUDIES

As in most modern sieges, the zoo animals were among the first victims in Leningrad. It was not a hard decision; what was the point of watching the poor beasts starve when they could nourish famished people for a few days? The hungry Leningraders felt not a whit of sentimentality as they slaughtered the animals, filling the cold streets with the steaming blood of tigers, lions, and giraffes. The zoo's livestock quickly disappeared as the people of Leningrad first acquired their taste for exotic meats.

It was November 1941. The people of Leningrad were beginning the Hungry Winter, the coldest winter ever in a city with a proud history of miserably cold winters. Hitler's army had surrounded them since September 8, 1941. The Führer needed to move the tanks and artillery that surrounded the city to other fronts, but the stubborn Leningraders wouldn't cooperate by surrendering. Hitler also didn't want to be burdened with the feeding of millions of famished Leningraders when the city finally capitulated. Hitler formulated an elegant plan, one that would both free up his artillery and reduce the eventual number of captives in his clutches. Hitler ordered that Leningrad be starved into submission. The siege would last 872 days.

After the zoo animals, the people of Leningrad next turned to their household pets. Killing beloved dogs and cats was slightly harder than killing zoo animals, but an easy decision nonetheless for hungry-enough people. The Leningraders had no choice but to supplement their official ration. The government gave manual workers an allotment of bread and cabbage that amounted to about 700 calories a day—about one fifth of an adult's daily requirement. Nonmanual workers were given only 473 calories a day; children, 423. Dogs and cats disappeared. Even the rats fled, as their food supplies disappeared in the city. Hungry Leningraders took some comfort in the knowledge that their rats now populated the relatively well-provisioned trenches of their German tormentors.

As the siege dragged on, temperatures plummeted to −40°F. The people collectively remembered that some wallpaper paste was made from potatoes. Wallpaper was stripped away from the living rooms and parlors of Leningrad, the paste scraped into pots and boiled into soup, a soup that tasted much more like paste than potatoes. Leather, too, could be boiled into a gelatinous mess that could briefly satisfy the sharpest pangs of hunger.

By 1943, as the siege entered its second year, all the animals, wallpaper paste, and leather had been consumed. The people descended into a rare kind of hunger, a hunger that tested even the most fundamental taboos. People began eating corpses. In most cases the flesh was still firm and well preserved by the frigid temperatures. The eating of the dead became a ghoulish fact of life, until inevitably, the hungriest began looking for fresher meat.

The children of Leningrad began disappearing. As rumors of cannibalism spread, it became illegal to sell any form of ground meat in the city, as the sources became too horrifically questionable. In one case, the bones of several dozen children were found inside the apartment of a concert violinist. Even his own five-year-old son was missing. The Leningrad police formed a special division to combat cannibalism. By the beginning of 1944, as even corpses and children became scarce, there were reports of people cutting off their own body parts and eating them in a desperate attempt to stave off hunger.

The Red Army broke through the German lines on January 27, 1944, and the siege was lifted. In all, a million Soviets had starved to death in that city—more than a thousand per day. People were forbidden, both officially and unofficially, from ever speaking of the cannibalism that took place during the siege. The Soviets had learned to a frightening extent how much the availability of food allows civilization to occur.

The Siege of Leningrad was just one, terrible example of hunger's role in World War II. The first starving survivors of the Nazi concentration camps were liberated around the same time the siege was lifted. Their skeletal images were just beginning to sear themselves into the public consciousness. Food consumption in occupied Norway had been near famine levels for almost the entire war. A hunger crisis spread across China as the war between Chiang Kai-Shek and the Communists wreaked havoc in the countryside; millions starved in 1943 in the province of Honan alone. Even the United States, with massive agricultural capacity and no battles on her own soil, saw shortages because of the war. The United States implemented nationwide rationing in 1942, transforming sugar, butter, coffee, and beef into luxury items. The American government, anticipating the Cold War, began taking a long look at the possibility and the implications of widespread starvation. They wanted the postwar world rebuilt in America's democratic image. It would be impossible, as Dr. Ancel Keys would often point out, to teach starving people democracy.

Those concerns were alluded to throughout the July 30, 1945, issue of *Life* magazine. Published during the strange summer that unfolded after Victory in Europe (May 8), but before Victory in Japan (August 14), the magazine seemed torn between an austere wartime stance and the ebullience of imminent victory. The Nazi surrender documents, signed by Nazi General Alfred Jodl, were reproduced in full. So were photographs of actress Ella Raines sunbathing beside her Beverly Hills pool.

In another article in that same issue, readers learned that there were close to three million "displaced persons" under the care of the Allied armies in Europe alone. Getting the DPs to the food or the food to the DPs was a major challenge for the fledgling United Nations. An editorial in that same issue of *Life* stated that Russia "is the No. 1 problem for America because it is the only country in the world with the dynamic power to challenge our own conceptions of truth, justice and the good life." According to *Life's* editors, Americans had to find a way to "equal the communist talent for persuasion."

Finally, in that same issue, framed by ads for Borden Milk and G&D American Vermouth, there was a four-page photo spread entitled "Men Starve in Minnesota." At the University of Minnesota in Minneapolis, readers learned, thirty-six volunteers were being starved so that science might understand the effects of severe malnutrition and how to treat it. Someone paging quickly through the magazine might have mistaken the emaciated volunteers for victims of the Nazi concentration camps, with their characteristic protruding ribs and empty stares. One man's grotesquely swollen leg was shown in a photo, the swelling an apparent side effect of the hunger. In another, several bony men ran shirtless on treadmills. Finally there was a stern doctor in a lab coat, the head of the study, who was measuring the chest of one gaunt volunteer, with large steel calipers. He was identified as Dr. Ancel Keys.

The photos must have provoked questions in the minds of thoughtful readers: Who are these men? Why would anyone volunteer to be starved? Have they learned anything? Who is this Dr. Keys? *Life* readers in 1945 had only scant captions for answers.

Ancel Benjamin Keys was born on January 26, 1904, in Colorado Springs, the only child of working-class parents. Two years later, his family moved to San Francisco where his father hoped to find work. They arrived just in time for the Great Earthquake. While their small house was undamaged, the print shop where his father worked was destroyed. The family fled to Los Angeles. Keys would claim all his life that during their refuge in Southern California they stayed with his uncle—silent film legend Lon Chaney. It made for an interesting beginning to an exceedingly interesting life story.

Keys' flair for drama may have been inherited from his famous uncle. His maternal grandparents, Emma and Frank Chaney of Colorado Springs, were profoundly deaf. Hollywood legend has it that their son, originally named Leonidas, learned his silent artistry by communicating with his parents via pantomime. It is highly unlikely, to say the least, that Keys and his parents stayed with Lon after the earthquake in 1906. Lon Chaney wouldn't move to California until 1910, and he wouldn't make his first credited film appearance until *Poor Jake's Demise* in 1913. In fact, at the time of the Great Earthquake, Hollywood's first film studio hadn't even arrived—the Nestor Company would open at the corner of Sunset and Gower in 1911. Keys was a two-year-old when he survived the Great Earthquake and subsequent fire—he can be forgiven if his memory of the aftermath was a little sketchy. It was the telling lapse, however, of a man who learned early on to like the idea of fame and celebrity.

Six months after the earthquake, the Keys family moved back to the Bay Area, to Berkeley, where Ancel would spend most of his adventurous boyhood. The Berkeley of Ancel Keys' youth was in most ways a typically idyllic small California town. Streetcars and automobiles still competed for space with horse-drawn wagons and strolling pedestrians. Gentle treeless hills rolled at the edges of the city. Inside Berkeley, mature trees and lush vegetation crowded the sidewalks. Trains connected the city to nearby Oakland, and ferries made the short trip to San Francisco. Ancel and his family lived in a plain, gray, two-story house on Shattuck Avenue, a street lined with similar houses crowding the sidewalk and each other.

It was not a religious household; his parents did not belong to any church. Once his mother did make Ancel attend Sunday school at the Presbyterian church near their home, but Ancel came away unimpressed. He did not believe in the miracles the minister spoke of, and he did not feel a great need for the comforts and promises that religion offered.

If Berkeley looked similar to other rural California towns of the era, it was different in one fundamental way: it was a college town. Berkeley was dominated by the University of California. No citizen of Berkeley could avoid brushing up against what was rapidly becoming the most respected institution of higher learning in the West. The histories of the school and the town were inseparable. The land north of Oakland that would become Berkeley was actually named by the trustees of the College of California, who had purchased one hundred sixty empty acres there in 1866 with an eye towards future expansion. They named the college town they envisioned after George Berkeley, an Irish philosopher who believed that nothing, not even physical objects, existed apart from perception. The entire campus moved from Oakland to this new city in 1873. Berkeley would incorporate five years later.

Ancel's father worked in a print shop. His mother kept house. Neither had a college degree. Their lack of education was in no way unusual. In 1920, when Ancel was sixteen years old, only 22 percent of the American population had an education beyond the fifth grade. Sixteen percent graduated from high school. A scant 3.3 percent had four or more years of college. In the college town of Berkeley, however, that percentage would have been far higher. A young, inquisitive boy like Ancel Keys spending his formative years in Berkeley would have seen higher education as a completely normal part of life.

If college was part of the background noise of Ancel's boyhood, so was a healthy and unusually varied diet. Growing up in

California, Keys regularly enjoyed a wide variety of fresh foods that were regarded as exotic or extravagant in the rest of the country, foods like oranges, olives, lemons, and almonds. Later in life, as he traveled the world, Keys would often complain that the diet of whatever city he was visiting was lacking in the fresh fruits and vegetables that he loved. In addition to the rainbow of foods grown in the region, California then, just as it is now, was an entry point for exotic peoples and foods from all over the world. When not enjoying his mother's highly regarded cooking, one of Ancel's favorite adventures was a trip into San Francisco's Chinatown to buy an egg roll and two bowls of chow fan for forty cents.

Keys was born in the same year that Teddy Roosevelt was elected president and he shared the president's fondness for the "vigorous life." He was not a completely uninterested student—at one point in junior high he even tried unsuccessfully to found a chemistry club. Ancel was just far more interested in exploring the western wilderness that surrounded him. At the age of ten, he and two friends fled school to live on Grizzly Peak, a hill that still offers wonderful views of the University of California campus. Keys and his fellow truants camped for three days, subsisting on dried prunes, bacon, and Aunt Jemima pancakes cooked over a campfire.

At the age of fifteen, Keys spent the summer working at a lumber camp. He returned home for the start of school, but soon grew bored again with Berkeley and the classroom. He left a brief note to his mother, and thumbed a ride on a car going south.

The ride ended in Needles, California, a Mojave Desert town that bragged of being the hottest city in America. Ancel couldn't find work in Needles, but heard of an unusual job opportunity across the border, on the outskirts of Oatman, Arizona. Hearing that the pay was good, he signed up.

Ancel was driven to the mouth of a small cave, an irregular horizontal slot that opened in a low desert hillside. He stepped down from the truck and followed the foreman a few steps inside. After the bright desert sunlight, it took a minute for Ancel's eyes to adjust. When he could see again, Ancel involuntarily jerked backwards as he realized that millions of tiny eyes were upon him, alertly staring to see who had disturbed their slumber. The ceiling of the cave, from where he stood into the darkest reaches beyond the dim light, was covered with bats. They were twitching, squeaking, and most of all, defecating. The floor was covered with their guano. It was ten feet deep in some places, reaching almost to the ceiling. The guano, the foreman told Ancel, was prized by fertilizer manufacturers. Ancel's job was to shovel the dry, odorless pellets into gunnysacks.

Day after day he filled sack after sack with his shovel, the nervous sleeping bats his only company. Each morning, a truck would arrive to leave fresh food and water, and to take away his filled gunnysacks. Ancel had only cold sandwiches to eat; there was no wood with which to build a fire. He dug a primitive latrine some distance away from his "bedroom," an old blanket that provided his only cover. At night, as he rested under that blanket, there was no light to read by, and nothing to read anyway. Every sunset, Ancel's day would end as the bats' work began with their frenzied, fluttering exodus from the cave. He stared at the stars until he went to sleep, vowing to learn more about astronomy when he returned to civilization.

Keys worked alone in the desert for three months, filling gunny sacks with guano and sleeping under the stars. One morning the truck came for his bulging gunnysacks, and Ancel got on too, and returned to Needles. He collected his accumulated wages, bought a new suit, a hat, and a train ticket, and returned to Berkeley.

His mother embraced him upon his return, curious about his absence, but relieved beyond any anger. Keys returned to Berkeley High School slightly more energetic about his studies than before. A lifetime in the college town of Berkeley plus a season shoveling bat guano had helped him see the value of a college education.

Unfortunately, his grades and frequent extended absences up to that point did not mark him as college material. However, a perceptive (or perhaps charitable) algebra teacher saw a glint of potential in Keys and wrote a recommendation glowing enough to gain him admission to the University of California, despite modest grades. He enrolled in 1922.

Ancel attacked college work with the same vigor with which he had shoveled guano in the desert. In addition to loading up on calculus, chemistry, and other science courses, Keys also studied German and Chinese. He worked thirty hours a week in the university library, and still made time to take his fellow students for thirty bucks a month playing bridge. He found himself in the running for the chemistry department's sole scholarship—and was greatly disappointed when he came in second to a student with a less challenging course load.

At the end of his freshman year, Keys took another unusual summer job. He signed on as an oiler aboard the merchant vessel the SS *President Wilson,* bound for the Orient. Keys' job during the voyage was to feel the bearings of the ship's two drive shafts and add oil if they felt too hot. Keys himself often felt overheated during his four-hour watch, guzzling gallons of water only to sweat it all out in the sweltering engine room.

The ship's first port of call was Shanghai, where Ancel was disappointed to discover that the Mandarin Chinese he had learned to speak in Berkeley was useless among the merchants on the docks. On a subsequent port call in Hong Kong, Keys discovered that the vendors could just make out his written Chinese. An excited crowd gathered on the dock to watch the foreigner haggle over the price of a small table in written Chinese. From Shanghai, the *President Wilson* steamed to Manila and Hong Kong, before finally returning to San Francisco. The voyage may have been Keys' personal introduction to malnourishment: he would say later that he and the rest of the crew subsisted almost entirely on alcohol.

Keys returned to the University of California upon completing his sea tour. Still stinging from the loss of the chemistry scholarship, disappointed by a B grade in advanced mathematics, and still burdened by an adolescent's impulsiveness, he resolved to leave the university as quickly as possible. He discovered that by taking the greatest number of courses allowed, enrolling in summer school, and changing majors, he could graduate early. He changed his major to economics and political science, and graduated with a degree after only three years.

Keys briefly charted a conventional course for his life. He took a management trainee position at Woolworth's. He even got married, to the beautiful and athletic Winnie Newton, a young woman he had met in school. But for the young man who had slept alone in the Arizona desert and taken the slow boat to China, the life of a Woolworth's manager did not prove adequately stimulating. After eight months of selling handkerchiefs and neckties, Keys quit. His marriage to Winnie would last only slightly longer.

At a crossroads, Keys sought out one of his favorite economics professors for advice; Dr. Paul Cadman taught courses on the history of economics and political thought. The professor somehow recognized that while Keys had excelled in economics, his true calling was in the sciences. He arranged for Keys to talk to a colleague, Professor Charles Kofoid, the head of the school's zoology department.

Kofoid, who had recently been awarded the Faculty Research Lectureship for his discussion of "Amoeba and Man," welcomed the promising young graduate student into his department. Even though Keys up to that point had not taken a single college biology course, he did not disappoint his new patron. By tripling up on his coursework and studying day and night, Keys received a master's degree in zoology in an amazing six months.

Keys' hard work was rewarded when he was offered an assistantship at the Scripps Institution of Oceanography in La Jolla, California, in 1928. After living on his library wages and bridge winnings for six years, the offer seemed too good to be true: one hundred dollars a month and a redwood bungalow on a beautiful seaside cliff. Keys happily moved down the coast.

The institute, originally named the San Diego Marine Biological Station, was founded in 1903 by University of California zoology professor William Ritter. It moved to its permanent location in La Jolla in 1907. The institute changed its name to the Scripps Institution of Oceanography in 1925, in honor of brother and sister benefactors Ella and E. W. Scripps. Although young, the Scripps Institute had already garnered an enviable reputation in the field of oceanography.

By the time of Keys' arrival, the Scripps campus consisted of a dozen or so buildings, the largest of which was the four-story library in the center of the property. All were within a stone's throw of the ocean and the institute's three-hundred-foot-long pier. Keys' bungalow was about a three-minute walk from either the swimming beach or the research boats. The house had no heat; none was needed in temperate La Jolla. It was built on stilts, and beneath it lived a benign family of skunks.

Keys' adviser at the institute, Dr. Francis Bertody Sumner, was an expert on evolution. He steered Keys towards a research project on fish survival in low-oxygen water, as it related to their number of vertebrae. The goal of the project was to demonstrate how a specific environmental challenge might affect the bony development of a species. The result was the paper *The Weight-Length Relation in Fishes*. In it, Keys disproved the nineteenth-century "cube law" that stated a fish's weight was directly related to the cube of its length. The study was also an early display of Keys' passion for meticulously quantifying the physical characteristics of living things.

Keys was able to turn his research into a thesis, one that he would take back to Berkeley to defend. On the way north, he stopped in Los Angeles to visit his uncle Lon Chaney, then at the height of his fame. Chaney's 1925 film *The Phantom of the*

Opera had made him a bona fide superstar. He was resisting the transition to talkies, a stance that was becoming increasingly hard to maintain in sound-crazy Hollywood. Lon also complained to his nephew of a persistent sore throat.

Once in Berkeley, Keys successfully defended his dissertation and received his first doctorate. Also, thanks to the glowing recommendation of Dr. Sumner at Scripps, Keys won a postdoctorate fellowship from the National Research Council. He would leave immediately for Copenhagen to study under the Nobel Prize–winning biologist Dr. August Krogh. Keys' academic star was now clearly on the rise.

Keys excitedly made the trip to Copenhagen in 1930, his first trip abroad since his stint on the *President Wilson*. After a long trans-Atlantic voyage, on his first day in Copenhagen, he saw an English newspaper with the headline LON CHANEY IS DEAD. His uncle had died of throat cancer during his journey.

Dr. August Krogh, Keys' host in Denmark, was not born into academia. He was the son of a shipbuilder, and would all his life display keen mechanical talent and a willingness to get his hands dirty. Krogh had studied zoology at the University of Copenhagen under Christian Bohr, whose son Niels Bohr would become a pioneering nuclear physicist. For an academic, Krogh was unusually skilled at designing, manufacturing, and successfully marketing medical devices. In many instances, Krogh's original research was made possible by precise instruments of his own design.

In 1923, seven years before Keys' arrival in Copenhagen, Krogh's rare combination of scientific acumen and pragmatism had him single-handedly bring a new industry to Denmark. Krogh's wife, Marie, was diabetic. During a trip to North America, the Kroghs saw two Canadian scientists manufacture small amounts of insulin by using a cow's pancreas. Krogh brought the method back to Denmark and founded a company to mass-produce insulin in this novel fashion. The company, Nordisk, rapidly became hugely profitable. Known today as Novo-Nordisk, it remains the largest producer of insulin in the world.

Keys soon learned of the professional conflict that led to the most famous episode in his mentor's career. Krogh, while studying the mechanism by which oxygen was supplied to the capillaries, came to dispute his mentor Christian Bohr's theories of oxygen secretion. Eventually, Krogh, using frogs and instruments of his own invention, proved that the capillaries opened and closed in response to their need for oxygen. While the study led to a permanent rift between Bohr and Krogh, it also won Krogh the 1920 Nobel Prize in medicine.

The August Krogh who met Keys in Copenhagen wore a goatee and pince-nez glasses that did not hide the twinkle in his eyes. His first question to the young scientist from America was "What do you propose to do in my lab?" When Keys stammered, Krogh suggested that he work on the "eel problem."

Scientists had long wondered how the salinity level in the eel's blood remained constant while they moved quickly between fresh and salt water. Dr. Krogh showed Keys a shallow tiled tank in the laboratory that he could use for his research. The next morning Danish fishermen delivered a slippery, black tangle of live eels. The rest was up to Keys.

The first challenge was grabbing an eel and fastening it to a board so that it could be studied. As the weeks passed, and his skill at wrangling the eels grew, Keys reasoned that only in the gills was the eel's blood close to the surrounding seawater. He suspected that the gills might be regulating salinity. The only way to be sure was to measure the sodium level in the water that was flowing out of the gills. However, measuring the salinity in such a small quantity of water was impossible with the standard analytical equipment of the day.

Working closely with Krogh, the master instrument maker, Keys built a highly accurate calibrated syringe. With it he was able to prove his hypothesis that the gills regulated the salt level in the eels' blood. Written with Krogh's encouragement, Keys' eel study became his first published work, in the *Journal of Biochemistry.*

One side effect of the study was a plethora of dead eels, the victims of Keys' dissections. Keys and the Kroghs' Danish housekeeper created a recipe for the meat. While Keys found the result palatable, he couldn't get his less adventurous hosts to try it.

Keys and the Kroghs grew fond of each other. In addition, Keys' professional successes in Denmark were encouraging. The flat landscape around Copenhagen depressed him, however, as did the gray climate and monotonous diet that lacked almost any fresh ingredients, eel meat notwithstanding. The language proved impossible to master for Keys, a man who spoke Chinese before he was twenty. He said that when spoken properly, the Danish speaker sounded like "he had throat disease." In 1931, Keys accepted a Rockefeller Foundation Fellowship to the University of Cambridge, and said good-bye to his Danish mentor. Knowing of Keys' unhappiness in Copenhagen, Krogh had arranged the fellowship with an old friend, Professor Joseph Barcroft.

Keys' new boss at King's College at Cambridge was a celebrity scientist in his own right. In one well-publicized study designed to research the effects of cold temperatures on the nervous system, Barcroft lay naked on a couch in subfreezing temperatures for an hour at a time, and recorded his impressions in a notebook. During World War I, Barcroft had put aside his religious pacifism— the Barcrofts had been Quakers since the seventeenth century—to work in the British military research facility at Porton Down. At the lab, Barcroft had disputed the claims of the French military about the lethality of hydrogen cyanide gas, a weapon the French had tested extensively on animals. To prove that it was not adequately poisonous for humans on the battlefield, Barcroft entered a gas chamber with a dog, and flooded the chamber with the gas. It killed the dog in under two minutes, but Barcroft strolled happily out of the chamber, having advanced science and his fame with one experiment.

By the time of Keys' arrival, Barcroft was studying the effects of high altitudes on human physiology. Advances in aviation during World War I had made high altitude studies a favorite of the world's more swashbuckling physiologists, each trying to outdo the other in duration and elevation. Barcroft began his studies on the subject by sealing himself for six days in a glass chamber in which the partial pressure of oxygen could be reduced to simulate the air at high altitudes. Barcroft sampled his own blood so often that he deliberately exposed the radial artery of his left arm for the duration of the experiment.

The pinnacle of Barcroft's high altitude work had been three months spent atop Peru's Cerro de Pasco from November 1921 to January 1922. One of Barcroft's published conclusions from that study was that permanent dwellers at high altitudes "are persons of impaired physical and mental powers." It was a generalization that incensed Barcroft's Peruvian colleagues.

Keys struggled at Cambridge to find his exact place in the world of physiology. He did little teaching and felt very much the outsider at the obligatory weekly dinner at King's College, where he found the food as bland and unsatisfying as the conversation. Even so, Barcroft took a shine to Keys. So much so that he campaigned for Keys to become part of the permanent faculty at Cambridge. To this end, Barcroft arranged for Keys to be awarded a PhD from King's College—Barcroft was afraid that the University of California doctorate might not be sufficiently impressive for his colleagues. The Cambridge doctorate, while perhaps more prestigious than the California degree, took considerably less work on Keys' part. It required no examination, no thesis, no work, and, in fact, no payment other than the cost of the elaborate mortarboard and silk gown with red stripes required for the graduation ceremony. Keys would keep the gown in his Minneapolis closet to show visitors for years.

Barcroft's efforts to retain Keys went unrewarded. In 1933, after only two years at Cambridge, Keys received a cable from Harvard University. Keys was ready to return to the United States, and a job offer from the nation's most prestigious university was the perfect opportunity.

Once at Harvard, Keys began planning an ambitious high altitude study of his own, in the spirit of Barcroft's work on Cerro de Pasco. Not to be outdone, Keys arranged for his expedition to go to the Himalayas. Keys organized an international team of ten men, including an Englishman, a Dane, and a Peruvian. The perennial political instability of the region had scared off other scientists, but not Keys, who somehow briefly secured the required permits he needed to scale the tallest mountains in the world. The spirit of international cooperation was not to last. The equipment was on a steamship bound for Karachi when Pakistan renounced its permission for the expedition, stating a crop failure in the region as their justification. It took all of Keys' persuasive powers to get the New York City longshoremen to unload his equipment on New Year's Day, 1935.

Undaunted, Keys immediately changed the team's destination to the north of Chile, to the site of a high altitude sulfur mining village believed to be the highest permanently occupied settlement on earth. Somehow Keys managed to get his team and his equipment to converge on a town called Chuqicamata. From there, they traveled to the miners' village, 'Quilcha, at 17,500 feet above sea level. The team formulated a scale by which they could subjectively evaluate their own relative acclimatization based on a number of variables. The robust Keys came out on top of this evaluation, scoring a 90 out of a maximum 100 points. The next highest total was 65, scored by W. H. Forbes of the Harvard Fatigue Laboratory.

Not everyone appreciated Keys' seat-of-the-pants methods and authoritarian style. At one point, a procedural disagreement with Forbes escalated into a full-blown fistfight on the mountaintop.

Keys' rough and tumble childhood served him well in the row, as he dropped the Harvard academic to the cold, rocky ground with a left-right combination. His authority over the expedition was not questioned again.

While the village was at 17,500 feet, the mine where the villagers all worked was at 19,000 feet. The miners walked an hour and a half up the mountain each day to get to work. In doing so they passed an abandoned village at 18,500 feet; the miners' refusal to live there, preferring the arduous walk, made Keys suspect that 17,500 feet must be close to the maximum altitude at which humans could live indefinitely.

Keys' own arterial blood would be an important part of the study. While they were not in the Himalayas, the sample he planned to take from his artery at an elevation over 20,000 feet would still be a record—that was important to Keys. So after months of planning and travel, climbing and acclimating, Keys found himself flat on his back on a frozen Chilean peak, waiting to give the record-setting blood sample.

He watched John Talbot, a young internist from Harvard, sink awkwardly to his knees on the rocky ground and fumble with his equipment. Keys wasn't worried. The minute he rolled up his sleeve, his arm went numb from the cold. He wouldn't feel the needle, no matter how clumsy the young doctor might be. Keys could tell that Talbot didn't feel well—the thin air at 20,140 feet affected them all differently. Keys had been up there with a graduate student acclimating for three days; Talbot had just arrived from their 17,500 foot base camp at 'Quilcha that morning.

Talbot found an artery after a few tries, and the two doctors watched Keys' blood bubble into the chamber. When it was full, Talbot stood and held the syringe in front of him.

"Well," said Keys, laughing, "is it frozen yet?"

Talbot's eyes rolled back into his head as he lost consciousness. For the second time in that expedition, Keys watched one of his colleagues crash to the ground. Keys realized immediately that

Talbot had severe high altitude sickness, a potentially lethal case. Talbot's face was blue not from the cold, but from cyanosis, a lack of oxygen in the blood. Keys leapt to his feet and called over the Chilean miners who had escorted Talbot to the peak. They carried him back down to the base camp.

Talbot fully recovered. In fact, he went on to become editor of the *Journal of the American Medical Association*. The Chilean expedition, despite its haphazard beginnings, was an unqualified scientific success, eventually written up in seventeen scientific publications. Keys' record for the highest altitude arterial blood sample stood for decades.

After the completion of his high altitude study, Keys returned to Harvard, where it didn't take long for him to again feel the urge to wander. He had no seniority at Harvard and didn't foresee any advancement in his near future. When he received an offer from the Mayo Clinic in Rochester, Minnesota, he took it. The clinic offered him twice his Harvard salary, a secretary and a technician, plus the opportunity to work "in a real medical environment" for the first time in his career. He arrived in Rochester in July 1937.

Few doctors then or now could turn down an offer from the prestigious Mayo Clinic, which brothers William and Charles Mayo had founded in 1889. They had learned medicine at the heels of their father, a frontier doctor and Civil War surgeon. They developed a revolutionary philosophy in medicine, that of cooperation between doctors of various specialties, with the best interest of the patient always the highest priority. In 1919, their practice had grown to the point that the brothers dissolved their own partnership and turned over all the practice's assets, including most of their own life savings, to a nonprofit foundation. The two brothers died within weeks of each other in 1939, shortly after Keys' arrival.

Despite the Mayo Clinic's hallowed place in American medicine, Keys found the atmosphere only slightly more stimulating than his stint at Woolworth's. After his years of globetrotting, he found rural Rochester to be "awfully provincial." He was disappointed to find that "all the docs talked nothing but doc business and the evenings were devoted to bridge."

He stayed less than a year. Lotus Coffman, the president of the University of Minnesota, asked Keys to come to Minneapolis and start a new institute, the Laboratory of Physiological Hygiene. Its ambitious if vague charter was "to try to find out why people got sick before they got sick." Keys accepted Coffman's offer. While Keys would retain his yen for world travel, he had found his permanent professional home.

The short stay at the Mayo Clinic did provide Keys with more than another recognizable entry for his curriculum vitae. While interviewing candidates for the chemist's job at the clinic, he met Margaret Haney. He not only hired her, he married her within a year.

Margaret was a native Minnesotan, from Duluth, where her father was a family doctor. Her mother was a descendant of Quaker refugees who had fled religious persecution in Wales. After graduating from all-female Wells College in upstate New York with a degree in chemistry in 1931, she found it hard to find a job, as did many in the midst of the Depression. She found her way back to Minnesota and a string of unsatisfying, short-term teaching jobs. When the Mayo Clinic called offering a chemical technician position in 1937, she jumped at the opportunity.

Thus began their professional partnership. When Keys left for the University of Minnesota in 1938, Margaret accompanied him, along with a secretary with whom she shared an apartment in Minneapolis. Margaret also assisted Keys in Mexico City, where he did a brief study on the heart sizes of children living at high altitudes. Finally, in 1939, Keys got around to proposing. They were married in a simple ceremony at her parents' home in

Duluth. Margaret would be at Keys' side for the rest of his life, both personally and professionally.

Keys' ambitious vision for the laboratory in Minneapolis soon took shape. The central theme of the laboratory would be, he wrote, "the exact measurement of human function and the factors affecting human performance and behavior." It would be, he thought, like a world-class engineering testing laboratory for the human machine. Keys was so bold as to say that he was creating an entirely new branch of science: "These are not questions of medicine or physiology or biochemistry or psychology or physical education, but invade and partake of all."

Keys' earliest work at the University of Minnesota had a novel sponsor. The school's athletic department funded research on the size of the hearts of athletes versus nonathletes. Keys disproved the folklore that athletes' hearts were bigger than nonathletes,' although they did pump larger volumes of blood and beat slower.

When he exhausted the limited research funds of the athletic department, Keys found a wealthier patron for his fledgling laboratory. In 1941, the U.S. military wanted to design a high-energy, portable, and nutritious meal for paratroopers. Keys took up the challenge. The work would gain for Keys a peculiar kind of immortality.

Prior to World War I, the military had not made an effort to manufacture different rations for different military situations. The foods allocated to soldiers were the same whether they were on base, marching, or in combat. The legislated ration for the Revolutionary War soldier was typical. He was expected to subsist for one day on 16 ounces of beef, 18 ounces of flour, 16 ounces of milk, 6.8 ounces of peas, 1.4 ounces of rice, and one quart of beer. The soldiers were expected to prepare the food themselves, an obviously difficult feat for a soldier on the march or under fire.

Throughout the nineteenth-century wars, the military evolved, and so did its ration. The ration of the War of 1812 increased the beef allotment to 20 ounces. In 1832, President Andrew Jackson horrified some career soldiers by eliminating the rum ration, substituting for it sugar and coffee. The Union Civil War ration added yeast. But while the exact amounts and variety of food items changed continuously, the military still prescribed the same foods for its soldiers regardless of the tactical situation they found themselves in.

This began to change with World War I. The innovations began with the "emergency" ration, a food package designed to be eaten in the trenches when no other food source was available. An emergency ration consisted of three small beef-powder-and-wheat cakes, and three one-ounce chocolate bars. All six items were packaged in an oval, lacquered can which could easily fit in a doughboy's pocket. The army's first attempt at a situational ration was an unmitigated success. By the time of the armistice, over two million emergency rations had been shipped to France.

The military also designed the "reserve" ration during World War I, a ration somewhere between the emergency ration and the full-blown chow line available to men on base. The reserve ration was intended to supply all the food an individual man needed for one entire day when the chow line was unavailable. The reserve ration consisted of a one-pound can of meat—usually corned beef—two 8-ounce tins of hard bread, 2.4 ounces of sugar, 1.12 ounces of ground coffee, and .16 ounces of salt. The total ration weighed 2.75 pounds, contained 3,300 calories, and was generally regarded as satisfying by soldiers in the field. The large, cylindrical cans, however, were bulky and impractical for a soldier on the march. Nonetheless, the development of a special ration for men in the field was a giant leap forward for military subsistence.

The army professionals responsible for all issues of supply and subsistence were the quartermasters. In the interwar period, the Quartermaster Corps made several improvements to the reserve ration. The ground coffee was replaced with "soluble," or instant coffee. The packaging was changed from cylindrical one-pound cans to smaller sardine-type cans. Pork and beans, a future military staple, was added in 1925.

By the mid-1930s, most in the U.S. military saw that war in Europe was again possible. The challenge of feeding millions of soldiers flung across the globe preoccupied military planners. In 1936, the army founded the Quartermaster Subsistence Research and Development Laboratory to develop new technologies for rations.

The emergency ration—or D Ration—received early attention. The value of such a ration had been seen throughout the first European war. The goal for the Subsistence Laboratory's designers was to create the highest possible caloric value in the smallest possible package. As with all rations, palatability was an issue as well. If it didn't taste good, the soldiers wouldn't eat it, and the entire effort would be wasted. The result of all these competing priorities was the "Logan Bar," nicknamed for Colonel Paul Logan, the head of the laboratory. It consisted of three 4-ounce bars made from chocolate, sugar, oat flour, cacao fat, and skim milk powder. The three bars were wrapped in aluminum foil and sealed in parchment paper.

The procurement of the Logan Bar directly reflected the United States' miraculous mobilization in World War II. In 1939, when Hitler invaded Poland and the threat of war began to loom, the United States Army consisted of just 227,000 men (out of a total U.S. population of about 134 million). By June 1941, six months before any official declaration of war, that force had grown to 1.5 million. By the end of 1942, the army had 5.4 million men on its rolls, and was procuring over ten million Logan Bars a month.

Updating the reserve ration was more problematic. The competing priorities of palatability, portability, stability, and nutrition proved to be a great challenge to the quartermasters at the Subsistence Laboratory. They soon began to focus on a six-can model—three cans of meat and three cans of bread. The final version consisting of six 12-ounce cans was called the "C ration," C for "combat." The ration would be steadily improved throughout the war. Chocolates and hard candies were added. Cigarettes were placed in the bread unit. Eventually the C ration was expanded into three meat units, three bread units, and an accessory pack containing cigarettes, water purification tablets, matches, toilet paper, and chewing gum. It supplied, in all, 2,974 calories and 114 grams of protein.

By 1941, it was already clear to the American military that the next war would require the extensive use of airborne soldiers, tank troops, and other small, highly mobile units. Even the C ration was too bulky for these kinds of strike forces. The problem was especially acute for paratroopers, for whom every ounce mattered.

Keys was uncertain why the army had contacted him about designing a new paratrooper ration. He thought it might have been some bureaucratic relating of his high altitude research in the Andes to the needs of paratroopers. Whatever the reason, Keys enthusiastically took up the challenge of developing the new ration.

Colonel Rohland Isker of the Quartermaster Corps went to Minnesota to help Keys get started. He explained the basic requirements: the army needed a ration that was small enough to fit in an army jacket pocket, but with enough nonperishable food to sustain a paratrooper until ground forces arrived and took over the battle—however long that might be.

Keys bought the first items at Witt's Grocery in Minneapolis. The initial ration contained hard biscuits, dry sausage, chocolate, and hard candy. Keys and the store clerk assembled thirty of the rations in brown paper sacks. Keys took the prototype to Fort Snelling, an ancient army base in the heart of the Twin Cities, where a platoon of soldiers was assigned to try the ration. As a result of the trial, Keys added gum, cigarettes, toilet paper, and matches. From Fort Snelling, Keys took the paratrooper ration to Fort Benning, Georgia, for more advanced trials on an entire company of soldiers.

While the nutritional specifications set by Keys stayed essentially constant, the exact contents of the ration were refined throughout the war. The final version, good for 2,830 calories, contained breakfast, lunch, and dinner, each packaged separately by the Wrigley Chewing Gum factory of Chicago, Illinois. Breakfast consisted of malted milk tablets, canned veal loaf, and instant coffee. Lunch contained dextrose tablets, canned ham spread, and bouillon cubes. Dinner was chocolate, sausage, lemonade powder, and sugar. Each meal came with a pack of four cigarettes. The emergency nature of the ration was reflected in its barebones nutritional content: each meal contained about 33 grams of protein and was slightly under the recommended daily allowances for vitamins. Other than the lemonade powder, the paratrooper ration was devoid of vitamin C.

But whatever its nutritional and culinary deficiencies, the paratrooper ration was lightweight, rugged, and compellingly convenient for military commanders. It soon attracted the attention of leaders outside the paratrooper corps. General George Patton demanded that the designator *paratrooper* be removed so that he could hand the meals out to his tank crews. The military obliged, changing the name to "K ration," in honor of its inventor.

At least, so goes the legend. As with much of Dr. Keys' work, this is not without controversy. At least two histories written within the Quartermaster Corps dispute that the *K* is for "Keys." Franz Koehler, in his 1958 book *Special Rations for the Armed Forces, 1946-53,* doesn't mention Keys at all in his history of the K ration. The Quartermaster School's official notes on the subject give Keys credit for writing the original specifications for the ration, but go on to say that "The letter K has no particular significance; it was chosen merely to have a phonetically different letter from the letters C and D."

The quartermasters' reluctance to give Keys any credit is perhaps due to their own long history of being underappreciated. The men of the Subsistence Laboratory were, like Keys, some of the early great thinkers on the subject of nutrition. Their ability to feed millions of soldiers around the world was a great and largely unsung contribution to the Allied victory. The K ration was one of their greatest successes. In 1944, its peak year of production, the army procured more than 105 million K rations. The very reason its name was changed was because of its great success and acceptance among military men beyond the paratroopers, its original customer. The men of the Quartermaster Corps might have been understandably reluctant to see any credit for one of their great achievements go to a man outside the Quartermaster Corps.

The K ration might have been even more successful than its inventor intended. Keys had designed a dense, mobile ration to be used for a limited period of time in extreme tactical situations. Army commanders, however, fell in love with the ration because of its durability and portability, and American soldiers across all fronts in World War II began to eat the K ration for breakfast, lunch, and dinner, for weeks at a time. The ration became hated, a victim of its own success and overuse. Interestingly, soldiers also became as fond of the K ration's packaging as they were tired of its contents. Ingenious soldiers used the ration's wax paper packaging as a drinking cup, a boot insole, and, since the wax was highly flammable, a means to start a decent fire, even at the dampest bivouac.

Despite the mixed reviews for the K ration, the army establishment had no problem in recognizing their effective young scientist at the University of Minnesota. Keys was named a special assistant to the secretary of war. He began attending monthly meetings in Washington, D.C. The army began directing more and more research his way, always with funding, always with the allure of helping achieve victory. Keys provided the army with a way to evaluate physical fitness in 1943. That same year he provided a report on heat stress. The K ration led naturally to studies on vitamin supplementation and deficiency.

Keys accumulated so much research hardware that he outgrew his lab. With the help of his friend and former patron, University of Minnesota Athletic Director Frank McCormick, he moved his laboratory to the ground floor beneath Memorial Football Stadium, the only available space on campus big enough to hold everything. The entry into the Laboratory of Physiological Hygiene became Gate 27 of the football stadium.

Keys also needed to find more room for his growing family. Margaret had given birth to Caroline in 1940. Henry was born in 1942. Keys and Margaret were for the first time feeling somewhat financially secure, so they took the plunge and bought a large country home on the shore of Lake Owasso, about fifteen miles north of the university. The lake was the site of swimming in the summer and skating in the winter. A massive outdoor barbeque pit that Keys built with the help of his father was the site of frequent entertaining. It was an idyllic place to raise a growing, active family.

In addition to providing Keys' laboratory with funding, the army also provided another hard-to-find commodity in wartime America: human guinea pigs. The army, through the Selective Service System, had a ready-made pool of healthy young men who could be part of the fun beneath the football stadium. They were the conscientious objectors of the Civilian Public Service.

The Civilian Public Service was the military's latest attempt at dealing with the troublesome issue of pacifist draftees. Most of these men came from the "Historic Peace Churches," a blanket designation that was more useful to the army than to the churches it identified: the Quakers, the Mennonites, and the Brethren. Early in World War II, the CPS mainly served as a means to hide these idealistic young men away in remote forestry camps. Keys would soon discover that medical experiments had become a favorite outlet for the altruistic urges of the more daring CPS men. Before the war, it would have been impossible to find large numbers of normal, healthy young men willing to suffer for science—for free.

The availability of the CPS men was a boon to Dr. Keys, a fortunate side effect of the war that he was not about to pass up. As long as he kept doing the studies that the army wanted, he could keep using the CPS guinea pigs.

With the help of the army and the CPS, Keys conducted an array of studies on the effects of various vitamins, both present and absent. He studied the effects on men of severe cold and severe heat. He exposed his human guinea pigs to excessive moisture; he studied the effects of thirst. In an experiment in 1943, Keys kept six CPS volunteers in bed for a month to study the effects of bed rest. He experimented on CPS volunteers with diets lacking in thiamine, riboflavin, and the B complex as a whole.

Keys became an enthusiastic customer of the CPS. He began to look to their ranks not just for volunteers, but for educated men to help staff the laboratory. One such man was Harold Guetzkow, a twenty-eight-year-old conscientious objector who had been working in Camp Wellston, a forestry camp in Michigan. Guetzkow had only a bachelor's degree in psychology, but showed promise to Dr. Josef Brozek, the Laboratory of Physiological Hygiene's chief psychologist, on his frequent recruiting trips to the camp. When Dr. Brozek asked Guetzkow to come to the lab to be his assistant, Guetzkow eagerly accepted the invitation to do something more useful for humanity than clearing brush and marking trails.

Guetzkow was in some ways an atypical CPS man. He was not a member of any of the Historic Peace Churches. He had been born in Milwaukee in 1915. His father suffered from multiple sclerosis. His family, desperate in their search for a cure, went to Europe in 1930 to learn about some new therapies. The battlefields of World War I were still fresh enough to make a great impression on Harold. The trip was unsuccessful in its search for a cure. Harold's father would eventually die of the disease. It was the beginning, though, of Harold's growing and deeply held pacifism. When World War II began, Harold was so sincere that he was the first conscientious objector ever to be recognized by his local draft board. He arrived at the Laboratory of Physiological Hygiene in late 1942, in time for the bed rest experiment.

Guetzkow soon became a highly esteemed member of the staff. Keys began to openly address him as a colleague, and credited him as such on publications from the lab. Guetzkow also served an important role as a liaison between the conscientious objectors and the laboratory staff. In this role he began to notice a growing morale problem in their corps of test subjects.

If the test subjects were in the beginning seen as a nameless, faceless commodity ordered from the Selective Service like test tubes from a catalog, that had changed. In addition to the natural familiarization that occurs with people who work closely together, Keys and his staff found very real scientific reasons to keep morale high among their volunteers. For one thing, a great many of their tests relied on subjective feedback. One of the advantages of using human test subjects was that you could periodically ask them how they were feeling and record the answer as part of the test data. Volunteers who were unhappy could skew the data. In the worst-case scenario, uncooperative volunteers could even give erroneous data, invalidating the entire test.

Guetzkow began to notice among the volunteers a growing uneasiness about the laboratory's close relationship with the military. Most had volunteered for the tests with the hope that their work would advance medical knowledge for all of humanity. Most of the tests they were participating in, however, were specifically designed for and by the military. The vitamin studies, for example, were designed to improve the contents of the meals for soldiers. The effects of heat and cold were being studied to help make soldiers better fighters in various environments. The frequent presence of uniformed army personnel at the lab reinforced the military objectives of the research. For many of the volunteers, as well as for Guetzkow, their work at the lab was beginning to bump up against their pacifist beliefs.

In 1943, Dr. Brozek and Guetzkow discussed the situation with Keys. The solution, it seemed, would be to design a study that would be equally attractive to the conscientious objectors, the military, and the broader scientific community.

After his work on military nutrition, it was natural for Dr. Keys to look for inspiration in the larger issue of world hunger. The war was taking a terrible toll not just on the world's food supplies; it was also devastating the world's apparatus for food processing and distribution. Keys had already studied the effects of specific vitamin deficiencies. Why not think bigger? Why not take on something as fundamental as starvation? A preliminary survey revealed that this topic had never before been studied in a systematic, scientific way. As he grew excited about the idea, Keys took it upon himself to convince a number of interested parties that such a study would be worth their sponsorship. Each constituency got a slightly different sales pitch.

Keys' primary argument to his military patrons was that solving the hunger problem effectively would be good for democracy. A famished Europe would be fertile ground for communist and fascist ideologues. Knowledge about hunger could be a weapon used to fend off the Red Menace. Keys had been attending monthly meetings of the War Department since the early days of the war. The inventor of the K ration knew these men well. The argument was effective.

To his scientific colleagues, Keys positioned the study slightly differently. Hunger, he argued, was an integral part of human history and was long overdue for scientific inquiry. He would eventually name the first chapter of his book on the experiment, "The History of Starvation." The first line of the massive work was "A full account of human experience with starvation would cover all of history and would penetrate every phase of human affairs." Keys noted accurately that the history of man is in large part a history of the quest for food. Yet almost no formal inquiry into the science of starvation had ever been performed.

In a kind of brute force demonstration of the prevalence of starvation, Keys compiled a list of 372 "Notable Famines in History" to bolster his claims. The list was broken down into "Outside India" and "Inside India" sections, so frequent were the famines in that country. The list was in straight chronological order, with just a geographic location and a year given in most cases. For a handful of famines, there was a word or two of amplifying information: "520 Venice, relief sent by Theodoric the Great." "1116 Ireland, cannibalism." "1574 Gujarat, plague."

Interestingly for an avowed atheist, one of Keys' primary sources for historical famine information was the King James Bible. He referred to famines in II Kings 6:26–29, Acts 11:28–30, and Genesis 12:10: "Abram went down into Egypt to sojourn there; for the famine was grievous in the land."

In the end, Keys' combination of national security, humanitarian, and scientific arguments was effective. The military agreed to let him use Civilian Public Service volunteers. The Historic Peace Churches all pitched in funds, as did the Home Missions' Board of the Unitarian Society. The Sugar Research Foundation and the National Dairy Council provided additional money. Keys even managed to get some funding for the experiment from his old friends in the University of Minnesota Athletic Department. Keys estimated the total cost of the experiment would be fifty-five thousand dollars—by far the most expensive research he had ever undertaken.

Over those next few days in 1943, Keys constructed an outline for the yearlong study. It would begin with three months of standardization, during which each man would be brought to a "normal" weight for his height and build. During this period the men would be fed a more or less normal diet. One of the main goals of this period would be to determine the number of calories necessary for each man to maintain his weight given a constant activity level, not gaining or losing—his caloric "breakeven" point. Another goal would be to establish baseline numbers for the multitude of tests that would be run on each man during the subsequent phases.

After the control phase would come six months of starvation. Each man's diet would be cut roughly in half. Potato and bread quantities would be adjusted on an individual basis such that each man's weight loss would adhere to the predictive curve that Dr. Keys had drawn, bringing each man down to an approximate 25 percent weight loss. The 25 percent figure was not completely arbitrary. It was an amount of weight loss Keys believed he could reasonably expect to achieve given the time constraints of the study. Keys also believed that while the 25 percent reduction would not cause overly serious health risks, it would be significant enough to effect meaningful, measurable changes, both biological and psychological, in the test subjects. Keys' goal for this period was nothing less than a complete cataloguing of every quantifiable change that occurs in a famished human being.

That would be followed by the three-month rehabilitation period, during which the men's recovery would be evaluated. The test subjects would be broken into subgroups to test recovery diets containing different amounts of calories, protein, and vitamins. This three months would be in many ways the real heart of the study. The point, after all, was not to learn how to starve people, it was to learn how to rehabilitate them. This data, Keys was confident, would be an invaluable contribution to the massive relief effort that was certain to follow the end of the war.

Keys hoped to begin the study in early 1944. One of the first steps would be to recruit volunteers from the CPS. He tasked Guetzkow with writing a brochure that would appeal to potential test subjects. Guetzkow wrote in the pamphlet that the experiment was a natural continuation of the conscientious objectors' heretofore thwarted desire to perform relief work overseas: "Every avenue of relief service has been closed to us, but here's something we can do now!" Keys himself continued with that theme in his section of the brochure, writing that knowledge gained from the experiment "would have practical utility far beyond the same amount of effort applied to any direct feeding relief." In addition to free tuition for university classes, volunteers could participate in a "school of foreign relief" within the lab, classes in language and health that would help the men become better relief workers, when that opportunity finally arrived. One potential apprenticeship for future relief workers was inside Minneapolis's artificial limb factories—"the largest producers in the world."

While the brochure took dead aim at the strong altruistic urges of the COs, it also mentioned the "intriguing possibilities" of Comstock Hall, the sole women's dormitory at the University of Minnesota, for those who wished to be "a guinea pig by day and a 'wolf' by night!" While the possibilities were no doubt intriguing to the men stationed in the monastic forestry camps, wolfish tendencies would be among the first casualties of hunger.

The brochure goes on for eleven pages, but years later, most men would remember only the cover. It was a photograph supplied by the American Friends Service Committee of three French toddlers examining empty bowls. Below the photograph, the brochure asked WILL YOU STARVE THAT THEY BE BETTER FED?

CHAPTER TWO

◄◦►

WORK OF NATIONAL
IMPORTANCE

URING THE AMERICAN CIVIL WAR, hundreds of Mennonites lived in the Shenandoah Valley of Virginia, the scene of some of the war's heaviest fighting. When the Confederacy drafted the resident pacifists, the Mennonites reported as ordered, drilled, and trained like good soldiers. Among themselves, though, they vowed not to shoot at another human being. General Stonewall Jackson said of the situation, "I understand some of them say they will not 'shoot.' They can be made to fire, but they can very easily take bad aim." Jackson decided: "I will employ them in other ways than fighting, but with the condition that they shall act in good faith with me."

The general's comments exemplify the complicated relationship that has long existed between pacifists and the United States military. While the military wanted the service of every able-bodied male, it had no desire to put genuine conscientious objectors in the trenches, where proselytizing pacifists would have been an unwanted disruption. The fact that genuine conscientious objectors made up such a tiny sliver of the population also made hiding them away an attractive option; alternative service for COs would not appreciably degrade military strength. Most generals concluded, as Jackson did, that the objector needed to be accommodated somehow. Hawkish politicians have railed over the years against alternative service, but the generals have almost always wanted to find a place for the country's pacifists equally distant from the front lines and the public eye.

The traumatic CO experience in World War I led directly to the formation of the CPS a generation later. The Draft Act of 1917 recognized only members "of any well-recognized religious sect . . . whose existing creed or principles forbids its members to participate in war in any form." The law required even those members to serve in uniform in noncombatant roles, such as clerical or medical duties. That requirement was unacceptable to many COs, who saw the donning of a military uniform as submission to military authority and a fundamental violation of their pacifist beliefs. The World War I law also failed to acknowledge members of religions that were not "well recognized" as being pacifist. One victim of this narrow definition was a draftee named Alvin York, from Pall Mall, Tennessee, a member of the obscure Church of Christ in Christian Union. He was ordered to basic training despite his application for CO status because the government didn't recognize his sect. During basic training, he was famously converted to the cause by a convincing commanding officer. Once in Europe, Sergeant York became the most highly decorated American soldier of the First World War. He once expressed perfectly the paradox of the patriotic American pacifist: "I didn't want to go to war. My own experience told me it wasn't right, and the Bible was against it too . . . but Uncle Sam said he wanted me, and I had been brought up to believe in my country."

In all, only 504 conscientious objectors in World War I completely refused to comply with the Draft Act; they were eventually brought before a court-martial. Seventeen of the men were sentenced to death, and 433 were sentenced to prison for an average of sixteen years. None of the death sentences were carried out, and all those sentenced to prison were released within two years of the Armistice, except for two who died in custody—one in Leavenworth and one in Alcatraz. It had been a horrifying situation for the peace churches, those 504 men, and even the army, which had no desire to create martyrs from the tiny percentage of the population that wished to reject combat. All sides agreed that if in fact the war did not end all wars, a better way would have to be found to accommodate conscientious objectors.

Despite the 504 courts-martial, there were some successes during World War I for conscientious objectors that set important precedents for the CPS in World War II. Fifteen hundred objectors received agricultural furloughs, a precursor to the "alternative service" of the CPS. A small number, eighty-eight, were even allowed to work overseas as relief workers for the American Friends Service Committee.

Between world wars, the peace churches steadily lobbied political leaders for a better, more comprehensive system. While no politician would be caught dead publicly embracing the cause of conscientious objection, military leaders were willing to listen to their ideas. The hard work of the peace churches paid off. The Selective Service Act of 1940 contained an objector clause slightly more inclusive than the World War I law. It recognized pacifism outside the Historic Peace Churches, pacifism obtained "by reason of religious training and belief," rather than narrowly accommodating only a small number of specific denominations. The act also allowed these men to serve completely outside the military system, performing "work of national importance under civilian direction." It was this clause, section 5(g), that authorized the creation of the Civilian Public Service.

The clause's vagueness would lead to problems. The men of the CPS would be unpaid by the government, and uncompensated in the event of injury or death. For those COs with families, the lack of pay was a huge sacrifice mitigated only by the case-by-case generosity of the peace churches. And as those men building sheep trails in the wilderness would soon find out, very often their work was of less than national importance. Many argued that by virtue of being subordinate to the Selective Service, a branch of government headed by a general, the work wasn't even under civilian direction. Still, the law was a major step forward for pacifists in the United States. It marked the first time that American pacifists during wartime did not have to choose between violating their beliefs and prison. The Historic Peace Churches quickly moved to take control of this new bureaucracy and give it direction. The result was complicated, messy, bureaucratic, and strangely effective.

As World War II began, 34,506,923 American men were registered for the draft out of a total population of around 134,000,000. Of these registrants, 72,354 applied for conscientious objector status, about one fifth of one percent. Twenty-seven thousand of these men failed the basic medical exam, saving the government the trouble of figuring out what to do with them. About 25,000 of the COs who passed the medical exam agreed to noncombatant uniformed service—the 1-A-Os. Many of these men became medics. (Desmond Doss, a devout Seventh Day Adventist and 1-A-O army medic, would win the Congressional Medal of Honor for his heroism at Okinawa.)

Slightly more than six thousand of the conscientious objectors refused to perform any kind of national service—most of these were Jehovah's Witnesses, who claimed that every one of their members was entitled to a ministerial exemption. The government disagreed. They were imprisoned.

Somewhere between the Jehovah's Witnesses and the medics were 11,996 men who, while opposed to any kind of uniformed military service, were open to performing some kind of alternative work. These were the men of the CPS.

As an organization, the CPS was created in the likeness of the peace churches. Each CPS camp—there would eventually be 151—was overseen by a designated church's service committee. The National Service Board for Religious Objectors, the group that ran the CPS on behalf of the government, was led by a committee of eight men, all from the Historic Peace Churches.

So what were the "Historic Peace Churches"? As far as the Selective Service was concerned, the answer was simple: they were the Brethren, Friends, and Mennonites. The history of the pacifist churches is more complicated. The Brethren and the Mennonites shared a common heritage. They were part of the Anabaptist tradition, a broad group of religious sects that arose in Germany, Switzerland, and the Netherlands during the Reformation. Like the pacifists of the 1930s, these radicals were heavily influenced by recent memories of a devastating war, the thirty-years war of 1618–1648. The term *Anabaptist* means literally "one who baptizes again," and it referred to the practice of adult baptism, one of the few practices that united the diverse sects. The Anabaptist churches were also adamantly opposed to state-sponsored religion. Consequently, members of the churches were often persecuted as being both traitors and blasphemers, causing masses of them to flee to other countries, especially the United States, seeking religious freedom. The Mennonites were named for Dutch Reformer Menno Simons, who founded the group around 1537. The Amish, a subset of the Mennonites as far as the Selective Service was concerned, were also named for their founder, Jakob Amman of Switzerland.

The splits, resplits, and divisions within the Anabaptist sects can be dizzying to outsiders. One of the starvation guinea pigs years later would talk about his father's dramatic split from the River Brethren, also known as Brethren in Christ, to join the Church of the Brethren, neither of which are to be confused with the Evangelical United Brethren. Such renegades founded the Anabaptist groups—and the churches have continued throughout the years to place a high value on individual interpretation and dissent.

The Society of Friends is a slightly newer institution than the Anabaptists and is English in heritage. The original Friends were followers of English preacher George Fox, who around 1648 began to teach a religion of "Christ within" and "inner light."

The term *Quaker* was originally a term of derision, referring to the spastic movements of Friends during their periods of individual divine revelation. Like the Anabaptists, the Friends believed in simple dress and pacifism. Unlike the Anabaptists, the Friends believed in enthusiastic participation in civil life. Consequently, many Friends became important leaders in the American experiment: William Penn, Thomas Paine, and Susan B. Anthony are three examples. Two Quakers have been elected president: Herbert Hoover and Richard Nixon. Quakers were also among the earliest and most consistent critics of slavery. Because of their longstanding commitment to be a part of the political process, the Friends were always disproportionately represented in the leadership positions of the CPS. The less worldly religious pacifists generally expressed gratitude for the political legwork the Friends did to make the CPS a working reality.

However, the Historic Peace Churches constituted only 58 percent of the CPS—4,665 Mennonite, 1,353 Brethren, and only 951 Friends. Overall, the CPS was made up of over two hundred denominations, with 673 Methodists the biggest group outside the Historic Peace Churches. There were also 149 Catholics, 17 Seventh Day Adventists, 108 Lutherans, 192 Presbyterians . . . and 3 men from a church called the "Fire Baptized Holiness." While the CPS program bore the unmistakable stamp of the Historic Peace Churches and would not have existed without their lobbying, it represented the complete, diverse, befuddling rainbow of American religion.

Even more surprising than the large non–peace church component of the CPS was the large number of men in the Historic Peace Churches who chose to go to war. Many religious pacifists saw World War II as a pure fight, good versus evil, and thought an exception to their church's peace position should be made. As the most worldly of the peace churches, the Quakers had a predictably large number of men who chose to join the fight. Richard Nixon, who joined the navy, is one famous example. The

Brethren, more worldly than the Mennonites but less worldly than the Quakers, are an instructive example. While the church is reluctant to look too hard even now at the number of their members who wage war in spite of the church's official position, of the drafted Brethren in World War II, fewer than 10 percent went into the CPS. Even the Mennonites, perhaps the most unified of the peace churches, saw almost 40 percent of their drafted young men choose to go directly into the regular military. CPS men from outside the peace churches would sometimes accuse the Mennonites, Brethren, and Quakers of having an easier time coming to a pacifist position, given the support of their families, communities, and churches. In fact, sitting on the sidelines during World War II was not that popular within the peace churches, either.

The head of Selective Service was Brigadier General Lewis Hershey. The fact that a general was in charge rankled some of the COs who thought they had been promised civilian direction. That General Hershey liked the CPS in large part because it kept the COs hidden from public view also bothered some COs, who resented his initial reluctance to allow them higher profile work. However, the general's support of the CPS was instrumental to its early survival. In arguing for the establishment of the CPS, Hershey explained to hawkish politicians the insanity of forcing the military to deal with thousands of uncooperative pacifists. Importantly, he also seemed to genuinely like the COs. He was born in Angola, Indiana, in the heart of Indiana's Amish country, and was a descendant of pacifist Anabaptist ancestors. He sometimes called himself the "Mennonite General." Lewis Hershey would go on to head the Selective Service for twenty-nine years and earn four stars, the only man in the United States Army to ever achieve that rank without serving in combat. Had he been a different sort of man, life for the COs in World War II might have been unbearable.

The early CPS camps engaged their men in work optimistically called "soil conservation" or "forestry." One starvation experiment guinea pig would say of his work with a shovel at a former

Civilian Conservation Corps camp in Lagro, Indiana, that it was "made work, and we were made to work it." Over time, however, the CPS began to find projects for its members that were important, daring, and sometimes even heroic. Two hundred forty men of the CPS became smoke jumpers, parachuting into America's northern forests to fight wildfires. More than three thousand CPS men volunteered in the nation's mental hospitals, and dutifully reported on the horrific conditions they found there. This venture into the medical field would lead naturally to participation in medical experiments. Dr. Keys was far from the only scientist to find a dangerous way for these men to spend the war.

The suffering of the CPS guinea pigs was the stuff of legend. Forty-eight CPS guinea pigs volunteered to wear lice-infested underwear in order to contract typhus. Other volunteers gargled the sputa from persons infected with pneumonia. Still another group strapped mosquito-filled boxes to their stomachs to contract malaria. The medical experiments satisfied some of the deep idealism held by these men; it allowed them to take risks and suffer for the betterment of their fellow man, all the while remaining true to their pacifist convictions. The medical studies also gave the Historic Peace Churches a rare opportunity to garner favorable press coverage in a nation that was finding most of its heroes on the front lines.

In all, more than two hundred men responded to Dr. Keys' initial call for volunteers for the starvation experiment. It was amazing that so many men would volunteer to suffer for a full year, under constant supervision, at no small risk—for free. Only the war, the Selective Service, and the CPS made it possible. It was a set of circumstances that was not likely to occur again. As he paged through the applications, Dr. Keys knew he could not afford to waste the opportunity. Picking the right men was absolutely crucial.

On a frosty Maine morning in 1943, Max Kampelman sat atop the ancient tractor and pondered again the ways that he was different from his conscientious objector comrades. He was not from one of the Historic Peace Churches that ran the CPS—the Friends (or Quakers, as almost everybody referred to them), Mennonites, and the Brethren. He was, in fact, Jewish. Jews were rare in the out-of-the-way locations favored by the Civilian Public Service. Jews who didn't want to fight Hitler were rare everywhere. Max was also a city boy, from the Bronx, while most of his pacifist peers hailed from farm country. On that morning in Pownal, Maine, Max confronted yet another trait that set him apart. The school for "feebleminded" children where he worked owned a small farm that Kampelman was to help tend. When they asked him to climb aboard the tractor to till the soil, Max had a confession to make. He had ridden subways all his life when he needed to get somewhere. He had no idea how to drive.

Being an outsider was a new experience for Max. Growing up Jewish in the Bronx, he said, "was like growing up Finnish in Helsinki . . . you met and knew only people like yourself." Although they met in America, his parents were both from the same Romanian town—Czernowitz. Their families came to America seeking economic opportunity and fleeing the endemic anti-Semitism of Eastern Europe. While fond of recalling the old country, they had no plans for returning. During the "Golden Age" of immigration into the United States (a loosely defined period starting somewhere around the 1846 Irish potato famine and ending with the National Origins Act of 1924), Jewish immigrants had the lowest return rate of any major group. Max grew up in a patriotic American household, where "here is better" was a constant refrain.

While memories of Cossacks and pogroms did invest a great love of America in Kampelman's parents, it also imparted a distinct antimilitarism that at times conflicted with their newfound patriotism. Kampelman's mother had made the long voyage to

America alone, as a despondent girl, after her beloved brother, a conscript into the Austro-Hungarian army, was killed in the First World War. Her mourning never completely ended. One day around 1930, the schoolboy Max came home and explained to his mother his latest all-American aspiration: he wanted to join the Boy Scouts. Upon hearing that her son would be required to wear a uniform, she burst into tears and made him promise that he would never join.

Max attended a demanding yeshiva school in Washington Heights that kept him and the other children of hardworking, ambitious Jewish immigrants in class until 6:00 PM, six days a week. Max excelled, skipped two grades, and enrolled in nearby New York University in 1937 at the age of sixteen. His father had died of a heart attack just a few months earlier at the age of fifty-four. The death was a severe blow to the family's finances, and it compounded Max's determination to succeed.

Like many young college students, Max soon opened his eyes to a new world of people and ideas on campus. In the yeshiva, all his teachers had been Jewish. At NYU, almost none were. Before NYU, Max had only known two non-Jews, one of whom was the Irish cop who walked a beat around the family butcher shop. At NYU, he met people from all walks of life. He took to the most liberal of student causes: labor organizations, social justice groups, and even the nascent civil rights movement. He became an enthusiastic member of the NAACP.

Max also joined the Jewish Peace Fellowship, an organization led by the Rabbi Isador Hoffman of Columbia University. The organization, in its "Statement of Purposes," said that "every war negates the fatherhood of God and the brotherhood of man." Rabbi Hoffman taught that Old Testament law demanded nonviolence: "*. . . and they shall beat their swords into plowshares, and their spears into pruning hooks: nation shall not lift up sword against nation, neither shall they learn war any more*" was a frequently quoted passage. Max's pacifism was heavily influenced by the leftist politics of his NYU classmates and professors. The Jewish Peace Fellowship convinced him that the pacifist stance was entirely consistent with his religion.

Max seemed to belong to every organization and write for every campus publication at once, while simultaneously holding down a dizzying array of part-time jobs and making fantastic grades. He wrote As I See It, a column for the NYU newspaper, represented the campus for the American Student Union, and joined the Law Society, all the while working in the bookstore and selling *New York Times* subscriptions, Fuller brushes, Realskill Hosiery, and Good Humor ice cream. He worked coat check at the dances for students more affluent and less shy than he, and took measurements for rental tuxedos on behalf of Rosenblum's Formal Hire. In his sophomore year he was elected president of the Menorah Society, a Jewish student group. In his junior year, he was elected president of the John Marshall Law Society. In 1940, in his senior yearbook, Max was voted not Most Likely to Succeed, but Most Ambitious. He recognized the ambiguity of the honor.

Max enrolled in NYU's law school in 1940, just as war began to look inevitable and the Selective Service Act was passed. Max's pacifism was already fully formed, a product of his family history, his religion, and his left-leaning student activism. He began writing for a pacifist newspaper calledd the *Conscientious Objector*. He continued to achieve academically with aplomb. In 1943, one year short of a degree, he took advantage of a recently passed New York State law that allowed law school students of draft age to take the bar exam early, with the understanding that they would still have to graduate from law school in the future—presumably after the completion of a military tour. Max was one of 265 New Yorkers to pass the exam in advance.

By 1943, the scope of Hitler's atrocities against the Jewish people was becoming known. Max even wrote about it in the *Conscientious Objector*. Max had a young man's un-nuanced confidence in his pacifism, though, and his early writings about the Holo-

caust reflected the shallowness that was the flipside of his idealism. After writing of two million Jews killed by Hitler, Max
wrote, "We'll never get anywhere for peace while national sover-
eignty exists." Max's decision to conscientiously object was similar in some ways to the decision of many young men across the
nation who were enthusiastically lining up to join the army, navy,
and marines. It was a decision motivated by youthful idealism
and some naïveté, a decision made with only the barest idea of
what lay ahead.

Unlike many COs, Max was also fully supported at home. His
widowed mother, scarred as a child by her brother's death in combat, was more than happy to see her only child spend the war in
what she thought would be relative safety.

Max registered for the draft like millions of other men in
America, conscientious objector or not. By 1943 every man in
America between the ages of eighteen and sixty-five was required
to register. There was no place on the initial Selective Service registration form for him to indicate his objection to war. His stance
would ultimately be evaluated by the local draft board. Local
boards were the backbone of the Selective Service System. General Lewis Hershey, the head of Selective Service, idealized the
system as being administered by "little groups of neighbors."
Because of the extreme localism of the procedure, objectors like
Max experienced a wide range of reactions to their position.

Once in the hands of the local draft board, Max's registration
card was placed randomly in a stack and assigned a serial number. The cards and numbers, as required, were displayed publicly.
In Washington, D.C., the numbers one through 9,000 were
placed in tiny capsules and then drawn from a large fishbowl. It
was the drawing of these capsules and the randomly assigned
serial numbers that determined the order in which men were
called before their local draft boards.

Max was mailed a questionnaire in 1943 when his number
came up—it was on this form that he had his first opportunity to

declare himself a CO. Those draftees who were calling themselves conscientious objectors were additionally instructed to obtain a special form from their local draft boards: DSS-47.

Max asked for and received DSS-47, which asked ten questions, some simple—"Give the name and present address of the individual upon whom you rely most for religious guidance"— and some philosophical—"Under what circumstances, if any, do you believe in the use of force?" Draftees were allowed to receive help in filling out the form, although Max didn't need it. Once in receipt of the completed paperwork, the local board passed judgment on each objector's sincerity. Each draftee was assigned an alphanumeric classification that was for millions of American men an introduction to the military's penchant for opaque nomenclature. Fully qualified draftees with no objection to war were classified 1-A. Objectors who could serve in noncombatant roles, such as the medic corps, were classified as 1-A-O. Objectors like Max, who would not serve the military in any capacity, were designated 4-E. Max's board, impressed by his intelligent arguments and obvious sincerity, approved his 4-E status without hesitation.

Not all draft boards were as enlightened as Max's. Some refused to provide objectors with the DSS-47 form. Other boards denied that there was even such a thing as a 4-E classification. One local board in rural Michigan was adamant that their patriotic county would produce no COs. Whenever someone applied for 4-E status with that board, they declared him medically unfit—4-F—to keep their region's record unblemished by conscientious objection.

Max learned that as an objector he would be joining the Civilian Public Service, an organization that promised him and the other conscientious objectors work of "national importance under civilian direction." His first orders were to a conservation camp in Big Flats, New York, where he spent his days stooped over tree seedlings. In his regular column, On the Democratic

Front, in the *Conscientious Objector,* Max expressed the frustration of many in the CPS when he wrote, "Selective Service prefers to have us plant seeds for fear that we may plant thoughts." It was a statement with which General Hershey might have agreed. Frustrated with the lack of pay, and the overall sense that the CPS was a form of involuntary servitude, a number of the more radical men in Big Flats began to contemplate forming a CPS union. They turned to Max for leadership.

Before the union could take shape, Kampelman read of an opportunity to work at a school for "feebleminded" children in Pownal, Maine. He had been at Big Flats for ten months, and he was hungry for a chance to do something more meaningful. He requested a transfer to the school and got it. The CPS union would continue its formation without him.

Between his tours of duty at Big Flats and Pownal, Max took time to attend the fifteenth annual conference of the War Resisters League in New York City. His brand of idealism without borders was on full display as he gave a speech to the throng of young pacifists at Nola Studios on May 27, 1944. Max told his rapt audience to keep the faith with respect to changing the world. "We will be in a favorable position for such efforts, for small as we are in numbers, we were the ones who refused to participate in the evil, we saw through the fog of artificial hysteria and kept our heads. We refused to be tied to nationalism. We remained true to internationalism. And here lies our strength." Max hoped that by transferring from Big Flats to a mental hospital, he would be one step closer to changing the world himself.

Max's choice to help the mentally ill was a popular one within the CPS. Men flocked to the mental hospitals both for the opportunity to do something meaningful and to escape the drudgery of the forestry camps. The institutions welcomed the men with open arms, since huge numbers of their low-paid attendants had fled for the greener, higher-paying pastures of the defense industries, and the motivated men of the CPS made ideal replacements. By the fall of 1943, one in six CPS men was working in a mental institution. Reform-minded conscientious objectors exposed abuses and made lasting changes in the way the mentally ill were cared for. The organization they founded during World War II would become the National Mental Health Foundation.

While in Pownal, Max was able to directly improve the lives of the patients in his care, even if he was unable—at first—to drive the farm's tractor. He soon began organizing trips for the patients into town. For many it was their first trip beyond the hospital walls in years. Still, Max found the work vaguely unsatisfying. Word of the Nazi atrocities weighed on him. Other people were fighting and dying to save the Jews from Hitler while he tended a garden and organized trips to the movies. Max remained committed to pacifism. Still, something didn't feel right. He was just too . . . comfortable.

Max was getting ready for bed one night in the CPS barracks in Pownal in 1944 when a new brochure pinned to the CPS bulletin board caught his eye. It read: WILL YOU STARVE THAT THEY BE BETTER FED?

Henry Scholberg's parents always told him that he was from Minnesota. As a child, the only life he remembered was in India. He was born in Darjeeling in 1921 and spoke Hindi before he spoke English. The jungle heat, the snake charmers, the bustle of the market place, the sad, averted eyes of the untouchables—none of it was strange to Henry. It was home. When his parents described the mountainous snowdrifts and the northern lights of Minnesota, now that was exotic.

His parents were Methodist missionaries, fighting a losing battle for Jesus Christ in a land long ago spoken for by Hinduism and Islam. His parents were also patriots—his father actually volunteered to be a draft official for the U.S. Consulate in India. It was a largely symbolic position, but it was one more link to the country their children had never seen.

It was an exciting time to grow up in India, and the impressionable Henry took it all in, much more so than his parents realized. They sent him to Woodstock, a Presbyterian boarding school at the foot of the Himalayas in Mussoorie. The school promised to shelter the children of Christian missionaries from the epic turmoil that was sweeping the subcontinent. It was a promise the school could not keep.

Much of the excitement surrounded Mohandas Karamchand Gandhi, the frail, unlikely leader who was devoted equally to pacifism and to India's independence from Britain. In 1930, when Henry was nine years old, Gandhi led the Dandi Salt March, which he concluded by manufacturing a small amount of salt through the evaporation of seawater. In doing so he was breaking the law—the British government held a monopoly on the production of salt. Gandhi vividly demonstrated the absurdity of the law while remaining true to his Hindu pacifist principles. Two years later, Gandhi began his "fast unto death," which resulted not in death, but in a pact with the British government to improve the treatment of the untouchables. Henry Scholberg had personally witnessed how nonviolent tactics could bring about concrete political change. The experience would stay with him his entire life.

One night in 1939, his senior year of high school, Henry and his peers were at the dinner table at Woodstock when the somber headmaster came to the head of the room and called for their attention. "Germany has invaded Poland," he told them. "The war is on."

Spontaneously, Henry and the rest of the seniors rose to their feet, executed a perfect Nazi salute, and broke into "Deutschland über Alles." It was a naïve gesture. Like many people, Henry and his friends had no clue about the true nature of the Nazis. They saw only that the Nazis were against Britain, and to be against

Britain was to be for India, for Gandhi, and for independence. It was a strange way for a pacifist to finish his high school career.

With high school complete, Henry said good-bye to his parents—without discussing his growing pacifist inclinations—and boarded the SS *President Taft* of the Dollar Line bound for the United States, a country he barely knew. On the boat, Henry met a stowaway who introduced the young missionary's son to the word *fuck*. Henry was amazed at the variety of usages his friend had for the word. It was just the start of his secular education.

In the United States, Henry enrolled at the University of Illinois in Champaign, in large part because his sister lived there. He majored in history. For four years Henry's student status helped him avoid the draft and a showdown with his parents over his pacifism. Even so, as a disciple of Gandhi, he was more than willing to take a principled stand. He considered briefly not registering for the draft at all and going to jail, but his worried sister and brother-in-law convinced him that registering would not be a violation of his pacifist beliefs, as he would just be telling the government his name and address. Upon college graduation in 1943, Henry faced the draft board and declared himself a conscientious objector. His parents, still in India, were horrified by the news but unable to influence their son directly from so far away.

After convincing the draft board of his sincerity, Henry Scholberg found himself ordered into the Civilian Public Service. His first duty station was an old Civilian Conservation Corps camp in Lagro, Indiana. There Henry discovered to his shock that not all the COs were as idealistic as he—one man bragged that he was "just waiting here until the war is over." Henry began to develop a certain snobbery about his pacifism, which he had cultivated on his own, without help from church or family. The boys from the Historic Peace Churches were expected and encouraged by their communities to avoid war, thought Henry. Their pacifism seemed easier than his, less authentic. After only two months at Lagro, Henry began looking for a more meaningful expression of his beliefs.

Like Kampelman, Scholberg's first opportunity to escape the drudgery of the conservation camp was a mental institution. During the train ride to Maryland, an uncomprehending Henry was propositioned by a homosexual, who told Henry that, like the COs, he "was a member of a minority group." It was yet another in a long series of eye-opening experiences for the missionary's son.

At the institution Henry and the other COs discovered that the staff seemed at times as disturbed as the patients. The COs called staff members "inmates with keys." The head nurse was a drug addict who would pass out during their regular bridge games. The superintendent was an alcoholic. After a year Henry was again disillusioned. He had wanted to do something important during the war. Instead, while friends of his were dying overseas, he was in a running card game with crazy people. But the lack of purpose was not Henry's major concern. After a year, he was deeply worried about his own mental health.

Henry was amused in his first weeks at the hospital to lose at checkers to an inmate who insisted convincingly that he was sane. Henry began to wonder, how could you really know? Surely his checkers partner believed just as fervently as Henry did that he was sane. A visiting nurse once mistook their chief psychiatrist for an inmate, another incident that amused Henry at the time, but it indicated how with the passage of time the patients became indistinguishable from their keepers. Henry began to suffer again from the terrible, barely remembered nightmares that had tortured him as a boy, when he would awaken terrified and sad in a remote Himalayan boarding school with no parent to comfort him. When he awoke terrified in the dark, he could hear insane, howling laughter all around him. Henry didn't know if the laughter was coming from the inmates, or from inside his own head.

In the summer of 1944, after eleven months, Henry saw the brochure. Will you starve? It was the chance he had been waiting for, the chance to act on his beliefs for the betterment of mankind, the chance to sacrifice. Most important, it was a chance to escape. He filled out the application and prayed that he would be accepted.

It was easy for Sam Legg to point to the day when everything changed: April 14, 1929. He was a boy, twelve years old, at his family church in Hackensack, New Jersey, his hometown. He was there with his sister. His mother was at home, having gone to an earlier service. His father was away in North Carolina on a short golfing vacation with friends. The Legg household did not take religion all that seriously—both parents were lapsed Catholics—but they did dutifully require attendance at the Episcopalian church near their home, and planned on sending Sam to the prestigious St. Paul's Episcopal prep school in Concord, New Hampshire, when the time came. Episcopalian was the right denomination for a family of their geography and ambition. Later that afternoon, in fact, Sam was to be confirmed into the Episcopal Church.

His family was solid, East Coast upper class. His father worked as a stockbroker in New York City during the day. His mother was raised in Grenoble, France, the well-to-do daughter of a glove factory owner. Sam and his siblings grew up speaking French as easily as English.

Halfway into the service that Sunday morning in April, when Sam's mind had wandered far away from the subject of the sermon and the holy mysteries before him, his aunt surprised him by touching him gently on the shoulder from the pew behind. He and his sister jerked around.

"You need to go home right now," she said. The interruption and the look in her eyes told them that it was serious; they rushed home.

Their father had contracted pneumonia in North Carolina. Their mother said he was dying.

Sam went into his bedroom and prayed far more earnestly than he had ever prayed in that ornate church that his father might live. For five hours he prayed as hard and as well as he knew how, blending an unschooled earnestness with what lessons he could remember from his recent confirmation classes. At 2:00 PM, the family received word that Sam's father was dead.

At 4:00 PM, stumbling through the ceremony in a dense fog of shock, Sam was confirmed into the Episcopal Church.

That was April 1929. In October, the stock market crashed, and much of the considerable wealth that Sam's father had accumulated as a stockbroker was lost. Most of what remained was squandered by a corrupt tax attorney Sam's mother had entrusted with the estate, a man whose gambling habit made him known at horse tracks up and down the eastern seaboard.

Despite the loss of income and the loss of a father, Sam's mother was determined to keep up appearances and send Sam to St. Paul's with what little money remained. It was especially urgent for Sam to succeed as his older brother had begun to drink and get into trouble. Sam was the family's last hope for respectability.

Sam failed the demanding entrance exam for St. Paul's. A substantial part of the test covered Latin, a language he had never studied. He was forced to go to a prep school *for* the prep school. After two years of remediation, he was admitted to St. Paul's in 1932.

Then as now, the young men of St. Paul's entered a world apart designed to meet the highest standards of New England's Anglophile elite. Their education came complete with cricket tournaments and Ivy League expectations. Sam never felt at home among the tailored greens and the rich young men of New England. He felt like a fraud, two years older than his classmates, with no money, no father, a Catholic pedigree, and an increasingly problematic brother back at home.

Like many lost, wounded young men before him, Sam found

comfort in religion. The personal revival that had begun inside him on the day his father died deepened in the face of the mandatory daily services and religion classes at St. Paul. While his schooling was Episcopalian, Sam's religious discovery was highly personal; he said that at St. Paul's "I got to know a fellow named Jesus of Nazareth." Sam's pacifism grew with his belief. To Sam, Christianity was obviously a religion of peace. The Sermon on the Mount, Thou Shalt not Kill—it was clear. He agreed with one of his heroes, Socialist reformer Norman Thomas, who wrote, "a careful reading of the New Testament certainly suggests that the burden of proof rests heavily upon those who would reconcile Christianity and war."

A campus event formally cemented Sam's growing pacifism. In 1935, St. Paul's received a contingent of pacifists who spoke to the students about the horrors of war and encouraged them to take a pacifist pledge. That staid St. Paul's would allow such an assembly was surprising, made slightly less so by the pledge's British pedigree. It was called the "Oxford Pledge," and had been born on February 9, 1933, when the students of the Oxford Union at Oxford University adopted a motion that "this House will in no circumstance fight for its king and country." The overwhelming support for the radical pledge—it was passed 275 to 173—shocked and alarmed the Western world.

Sam Legg listened to the speakers and read the pledge that was written on a huge placard behind the speaker's platform. The Americanized version had replaced "king and country" with a refusal to "support the government of the United States in any war it might undertake." It seemed a fair summary of the pacifism he got from the Bible, a logical complement to Thou Shalt not Kill. The speakers repeated the pledge, praised it, and in the end, all the St. Paul's boys present took it, vowing never to fight.

The Oxford Movement was the most visible manifestation of a vigorous peace movement that had been sweeping across both sides of the Atlantic during the 1930s, fueled by memories of the

Great War and books like *All Quiet on the Western Front* and *A Farewell to Arms*. The movement of the 1930s was of such magnitude that American military leaders were concerned about manpower shortages in future wars—a national poll conducted in 1933 found that 39 percent of American college students supported the Oxford Pledge. The military men need not have been concerned. Even before World War II, when the Spanish Civil War broke out, students on the left abandoned their pacifism and suddenly demanded the military service of every able-bodied student radical. It was an illustration of the truism authored by Colman McCarthy years later, that being a pacifist between wars is as easy as being a vegetarian between meals. By the time World War II began, the nation's corps of conscientious objectors contained only a very small group of men like Legg who had taken the Oxford Pledge and had taken it seriously.

Sam managed to get through his four years at St. Paul's with decent grades. To him and the other graduating seniors, there were only three colleges worth considering: Harvard, Yale, and Princeton. Sam conducted a brief survey of his peers, and upon discovering that most of the kids he liked the least were going to Harvard, he applied to Yale, and was accepted.

He chose to major in French although fluent in the language before setting foot in New Haven. He needed every advantage because he spent less than half his time on campus. His brother back in Hackensack had fathered two children whom he was not supporting, and his frantic mother frequently asked the dutiful Sam to help. Sam graduated from Yale with his degree in French in 1940. He was invited by the head of his department to pursue a doctorate, but Sam's complicated family situation made that impossible.

Sam got a teaching job close to Hackensack, where he could support his mother and bail out his brother. He dutifully registered for the draft as a conscientious objector, but in May 1941 was drafted A-1, the most eligible category, because of a bureaucratic error. Sam called the draft board and explained, and they graciously allowed him to complete the school year and even take his mother on a New England tour early in the summer. Sam finally entered the Civilian Public Service in August 1941 and was sent to a Quaker camp in Buck Creek, Pennsylvania, where he and hundreds of other COs helped build the Blue Ridge Parkway with spade and shovel. He would be in the Buck Creek barracks listening to the New York Philharmonic on the radio when the broadcast was interrupted by news of the attack on Pearl Harbor.

After nine months in Buck Creek, Sam transferred to Coleville, California, where he helped build a "sheep trail" with hand tools. Sheep clearly didn't need trails: the curious animals wandered among the COs as they worked. Sam asked the superintendent, a forest ranger openly hostile to the COs, if they could use some of the earthmoving equipment parked around their camp to build the trail.

"Son," said the ranger, "if we use that equipment, we'll finish this trail in two hours, and then what will I do with all of you?"

When not building trails for unappreciative sheep, Sam and the others helped fight fires, a more exciting and gratifying activity. They fought the blazes on foot, with shovels, axes, and backpacks equipped with nozzles and a can holding forty pounds of water to spray on the flames.

After a year of hard labor in Coleville, Sam received exciting news. It appeared that the men of the CPS might actually be allowed to perform relief work overseas. It was something that they had heard rumors about since joining the CPS; now it was happening. Sam immediately applied for and was accepted into the one-year training program for relief workers at Swarthmore, a Quaker college in Pennsylvania.

The curriculum included classes entitled World Relief Needs, Community Nutrition, Community Hygiene, and orientation classes on Central Europe, South America, and China. It was an exciting time, as Sam and the others contemplated where they might go and the good they might do for their fellow man. The government had somehow accommodated their pacifist beliefs in a way that would allow them to directly serve the suffering victims of war. Within a few months, the group at Swarthmore heard that a Mennonite CPS unit was actually en route to China to begin relief work.

The elation was short-lived. Congressman Joseph Starnes of Alabama, whose son was fighting in the Pacific Theater, was indignant that government money would be used to ensconce these slackers in a cushy school while good young American boys were spilling their blood overseas. He attached a rider to the War Department appropriation bill of January 1943 prohibiting the use of government money to send COs overseas.

The dream of real relief work died. The Mennonite unit en route to China was recalled, the college relief work courses were closed, and Sam Legg was sent from Swarthmore to the soil conservation camp in Big Flats, New York. Sam went back to shoveling, chopping, and sinking deeper into despair. The CPS work now truly seemed like a prison sentence. Like many of the others, Sam had always resented the fact that the CPS men weren't paid by the government for their work, although the peace churches did pitch in to give them $2.50 a month. The men were housed and fed, in the fashion of Depression-era work programs, but in most cases they had to provide even their own clothing. Sam's resentment grew when he learned that German POWs received eighty cents per day for their labor. (Men killed or disabled in the CPS would also go uncompensated. In all, 1,500 COs with disabilities were discharged without pay from the CPS, and 30 died in the camps—for reasons ranging from heart failure to being crushed in a feed grinder.)

In early 1944, Sam received another opportunity to do something more useful than chop wood. The CPS was sending men to a mental hospital in New Lisbon, New Jersey. Although not quite as glamorous as the overseas relief work, it was better than soil conservation. Sam volunteered and was accepted.

Like other COs before him, Sam found the work in the mental hospital challenging but gratifying. After his experiences with the hostile ranger in Coleville, he was pleasantly surprised that the administration actually listened when he and the other COs made suggestions about how to run the ward. He was close enough to home to comfort his increasingly needy mother and bail out his increasingly problematic brother. He was just starting to get comfortable in New Lisbon when the assistant director, fellow CO Marshall Sutton, presented him with a brochure that asked him if he would starve.

CHAPTER THREE

THE CORNELIUS RHOADS AWARD

D R. KEYS DISPATCHED Drs. Henry Longstreet Taylor, Josef Brozek, Austin Henschel, and Harold Guetzkow to CPS camps around the country. They interviewed the volunteers, performed a cursory medical exam, and asked the men about their health. They also reviewed the Selective Service health record of each candidate. Men whose weight varied greatly from the norm were dismissed, as were husbands. Keys warned knowingly that married life inevitably interfered "with the maintenance of controlled conditions." Keys gruffly summarized one of the goals of the initial screening as the elimination of "all the kooks."

Keys' actual criteria were slightly more specific. Good physical health was one of four broad requirements. To assess physical health, Keys had the results of the initial physical exam plus the data contained in each volunteer's Selective Service medical record. Keys recognized that in selecting only healthy men, he was explicitly not recreating the famine conditions of Europe, where the hungry often had serious health conditions complicating their starvation. Keys accepted this—also unlike in the war zone, his test subjects would be able to go to sleep at night without having to worry about bombs falling on their beds. Dr. Keys' goal was not to recreate a famine-stricken, war-ravaged Europe, but to scientifically isolate and study the effects of hunger. For that, Keys needed strong, healthy men whose bodies would yield data for him for an entire year.

Sound mental health was a second, more elusive criterion. For this, Keys relied heavily on a relatively new clinical tool: the Minnesota Multiphasic Personality Inventory. Every applicant took it.

The MMPI had been published just the year before, in 1943, by two of Dr. Keys' University of Minnesota colleagues: Drs. Starke Hathaway and J. C. McKinley. To take the MMPI, each subject was given a stack of 550 cards. Each card had a statement on it such as "I am happy most of the time" or "What others think does not bother me." The test subject placed each card onto a true, false, or "cannot say" pile. The answers of the test subjects were compared to those of persons known to be suffering from a variety of "reasonably clear-cut psychiatric syndromes," such as hypochondria, depression, schizophrenia, and paranoia. The innovation of the MMPI was that the answers of the subjects had no inherent meaning in and of themselves—only in how they compared to the answers of those with known mental conditions. The data for each man was charted on a graph with nine variables (each representing one of the clear-cut syndromes) as well as placed on a masculinity-femininity scale.

The MMPI of one of the more promising candidates caught Keys' attention. Henry Scholberg's profile showed a pronounced elevation in the "psychotic" end—the hypochondria, depression, and hysteria scales. What's more, Henry admitted in interviews that he sometimes questioned his own mental health, especially during his sojourn in Maryland. During his lonely days at the boarding school in India, he had been plagued by nightmares. At the University of Illinois, a school psychiatrist had told Henry that he was "a mess." While Dr. Keys liked the apparent objectivity of the MMPI, he also carefully considered the feedback received for each candidate from the CPS camp directors. Henry Scholberg's peers and supervisors all said that he was a dedicated, personable young man, one they could depend on. Keys pondered Henry's record, along with a hundred others.

The third criterion set by Keys for screening volunteers was a demonstrated ability to get along well with others under trying conditions. For this, Keys again relied heavily on the input of the individual camp directors. He knew the starvation experiment would be no place for the short-tempered or the thin-skinned, and carefully sought to eliminate such men from consideration.

Finally, Keys wanted to enlist only those men who had a genuine interest in relief and rehabilitation. He believed the full motivation of the test subjects was most likely if the subjects had "a personal sense of responsibility in bettering the nutritional status of famine victims." He knew that many in the CPS had been frustrated by their inability to work overseas directly with the victims of war. He wanted volunteers who believed the starvation experiment would be an enterprise just as valuable and noble.

Dr. Keys' staff members brought back to Minneapolis the file of each man who successfully completed the initial screening. At a senior staff meeting, the file of each was evaluated. Forty men were deemed to meet all the requirements. They were brought to Minneapolis for a final screening. Thirty-six of these were finally invited to participate in the experiment. They included Sam Legg, Max Kampelman, and Henry Scholberg. Dr. Keys hoped his careful selection process had yielded a group of men tough enough to endure the entire twelve months.

Before they even began, Keys cautioned each man about the potential dangers of the experiment, although only in the most general terms, as no one knew what the exact dangers were. Reduced immunity to infectious diseases was assumed. Diabetes, the volunteers learned, was "intimately related to the nutritional state." There was even the concept of a lethal level of weight loss, said to be around 40 percent by a German scientist named Krieger in 1921. While Keys said that that concept should be "relegated to the rich store of scientific mythology," it had enough believers that Keys felt compelled to address it.

Tuberculosis was held out as one of the gravest risks to the men. The disease had for centuries been associated with famine, although the exact mechanism of the link had so far eluded scientists. For men of the subjects' generation, the thought of tuberculosis had the same terrifying resonance polio would have in the years after the war. Caused by the *Mycobacterium tuberculosis,* the disease caused fever, night sweats, bloody coughing, and general deterioration often leading to death. As it seemed to consume the body from within, the disease was still often referred to by its cruder, more descriptive alias, "consumption." As the disease was highly contagious, society's answer to it had been to build sanitariums in the countryside where tuberculosis sufferers could either recover or die in isolation.

While it was reasonable to expect that none of the men would be exposed to tuberculosis during the experiment, as a precaution all had their chest X-rays examined for the characteristic lesions of TB, and all were given the Mantoux Test, in which a small injection of the bacteria was given to check for a reaction. The men were also asked if they had ever been exposed to the disease. No volunteer at risk for TB could be accepted.

Interestingly, Keys learned as he surveyed the links between hunger and disease, there was one class of illness for which folklore held out starvation as a potential cure: cancer. Since the Middle Ages, fasting had been prescribed as a treatment for tumors and swellings. While Keys criticized the scientific literature on the subject as "overburdened with far more conclusions than facts," he acknowledged that there seemed to be some basis for the claim. Cancer did appear in lower frequency among undernourished populations of laboratory animals. Keys suggested that the "high metabolic demands of neoplastic tissues" might make it so, and he went on to write that "dietary restrictions, perhaps coupled with increased physical activity, may be beneficial in cancer control."

Physically, the thirty-six men selected closely resembled their draftee peers. They were on average 25.5 years old, the youngest being Richard Mundy, a twenty-year-old Baptist from Bloomington, Indiana, and the oldest being thirty-three-year-old Philip Liljengren, a member of the Evangelical Mission Covenant church in Chicago. They weighed on average 152.7 pounds, and were 5 feet 10 inches tall. (By twenty-first-century American standards, these men, who came of age during the Depression, did not have much weight to lose. While the average American male is still 5 feet 10 inches, his average weight has risen to 169.6 pounds.) The measurements revealed that the men were slightly thinner for their height than the population at large.

Intellectually and educationally, the men bore less similarity to their peers in the army. Every one of the test subjects had at least one year of college; eighteen had college degrees. The Thorndike CAVD (completion, arithmetic, vocabulary, and directions) Test, an early IQ test, also showed the men to be intellectually well above average. In fact, as Dr. Keys was proud to point out, their average score on the CAVD—426—surpassed that of the Masters of Arts candidates at the teacher's college of Columbia University. On the army's own intelligence test, the Army General Classification Test, the candidates scored about two complete standard deviations higher than the average Selective Service inductee.

As for the psychological profiles, the scores of the men on the MMPI fell squarely within the average ranges for men of their age. The scores did skew slightly towards the "feminine" end of the MMPI, a fact Dr. Keys attributed to the higher than average interest of his group in "cultural activities."

Of course, the religious beliefs of the men set them apart from America's soldiers in a fundamental way. The religious affiliations of the men selected did not quite mirror those of the CPS either. The Brethren were overrepresented in Dr. Keys' laboratory. While they made up about 11 percent of the CPS, they made up the single biggest group in the lab—nine men out of thirty-six, or 25 percent of the guinea pigs. Overall, the non–Historic Peace Churches were overrepresented in the lab, accounting for 21 of the 36 guinea pigs, or 58 percent. The biggest group from the non-HPCs were Henry Scholberg and his fellow Methodists, with five representatives, tying the Friends in their participation.

The most glaring statistical disparity was in the group's lack of Mennonites. The Mennonites made up the single largest religious group in the CPS—4,665 men, or about 39 percent of the CPS overall. They sent, however, only one man into the starvation experiment. One possible explanation for this was that the Mennonite CPS camps were known for being the most cohesive, least diverse, and most religiously devout camps in the CPS. Perhaps the Mennonite men did not on the whole feel the desperate need to explore options away from the camps in the way that men like Scholberg and Kampelman did.

As with the CPS as a whole, the Historic Peace Churches would receive almost all of the credit for the starvation experiment, despite making up less than half the volunteers. Even the normally meticulous Ancel Keys would get it wrong when he wrote about the experiment in 1999, stating that other than Max Kampelman, "almost all of the other subjects were Quakers, Mennonites, or members of the Church of the Brethren." Americans had an easy time accepting pacifism from these small, curious churches. Pacifists from "normal" American churches were harder to understand, and often conveniently forgotten, even by those closest to the Civilian Public Service.

Dr. Keys did little soul searching about the morality of using human test subjects. Indeed, in his writing on the subject, he viewed the availability of the CPS subjects as nothing less than a great stroke of fortune. Keys was not out of the mainstream of medical thought in this regard. In fact, he was part of a long tradition of conducting research on humans. For most of history, it has been regarded as common sense that to learn how to treat humans, you must conduct research on humans. Dr. Keys would only have been surprised had he known how fundamentally that assumption was about to change.

Research that by today's standards would be condemned as categorically unethical has led to some of medicine's greatest triumphs. In 1721, Zabdiel Boylston of Brookline, Massachusetts, scratched his own son with the pus of an infected smallpox sore to test a piece of folklore about the disease. Boylston was the son of a doctor, but had no formal training of his own. The theory he was testing came from slaves, who reportedly immunized themselves against smallpox in a similar way. Boylston's son became slightly sick, but recovered, and was immune to the dreaded disease from then on.

Boylston's theory was not without critics. Religious zealots fought the practice of inoculation as unnatural and contrary to the will of God. Boylston went on to immunize hundreds of others anyway, and to publish the results of his work. While his mortality rate of 2 percent would be unacceptable in any modern clinical trial, the efficacy of Boylston's work was soon widely accepted.

Dr. Keys wasn't the first to experiment on humans on behalf of the United States military either. Dr. Walter Reed was tasked with finding a cure for yellow fever in 1900. Reed was the wunderkind son of a Methodist minister, and at eighteen, the youngest graduate ever from the University of Virginia Medical School. He had distinguished himself in 1898 on the army's Typhoid Board, and was a natural choice to lead the charge against the scourge of yellow fever.

The disease had plagued the South for two hundred years. It began with chills and a headache, followed by pains in the arms, legs, and back. A fever stage was then accompanied by jaundice, giving the disease its name. Finally, after a "stage of calm," the disease returned to finish its work, with severe fever, internal bleeding, and black vomit. The mortality rate ranged from 40 percent to, as Napoleon found out when the disease wiped out his expeditionary force in 1802, as high as 90 percent. The fever had killed more soldiers in the Spanish-American War than enemy fire, stopped French efforts on the Panama Canal, and was a major factor in influencing Napoleon to sell the fever-riddled Louisiana Purchase to Thomas Jefferson in 1803.

To attack the disease, Reed traveled to Cuba. There he deliberately exposed Spanish volunteers to mosquitoes to test the unpopular thesis that the insects transmitted yellow fever. Reed had other test subjects sleep on the bedding of infected men and wear their clothing to disprove the commonly held belief that the disease was transmitted in that way. Dr. Reed's test protocols were enlightened for the era. Not only did he fully inform his test subjects in writing about the known risks, he paid them: one hundred dollars if they didn't contract the illness, and two hundred dollars if they did. Reed's research proved the culpability of the mosquitoes and saved countless lives.

Many test subjects through the ages didn't fare as well as Reed's Spaniards. While researching cancer in Puerto Rico in 1931, Dr. Cornelius Rhoads saw thirteen patients die under his care. While he was cleared of any wrongdoing at the time, a letter was found on his desk by a lab technician late that year. In it, Dr. Rhoads described Puerto Ricans as "the dirtiest, laziest, most degenerate and thievish race of men to inhabit this sphere . . . What the island needs is not public health work but a tidal wave or something to totally exterminate the population. I have done my best to further the process of extermination by killing off eight and transplanting cancer into several more."

The letter caused a furor. Rhoads, who had already beaten a hasty retreat to New York by the time the letter was publicized, argued unconvincingly that the letter was a "fantastic and playful composition written entirely for my own diversion and intended as parody." Puerto Rican nationalists held the letter up as proof of the genocidal intentions of the American occupiers. Almost twenty years later, when two Puerto Rican militants attempted to assassinate President Harry Truman, they cited the letter as one of their justifications.

Rhoads' colleagues in the medical profession were more forgiving. He served as chief of the medical department of the army's chemical warfare division during World War II, and won the Legion of Merit for his efforts. After the war, he became director of Memorial Hospital in New York, where he pioneered chemotherapy by using mustard gas on malignant tumors. Rhoads won the Clement Cleveland Medal from the New York Cancer Committee in 1948 and the American Cancer Society Award in 1955. Rhoads became the first director of the Sloan-Kettering Institute for Cancer Research, and remained in that position until his death in 1959. Until 2003, the American Association for Cancer Research named its annual prize for most promising young cancer researcher the Cornelius P. Rhoads Memorial Award.

As Dr. Keys began the Starvation Experiment, the atrocities of the Nazi doctors were just becoming known—the attendant outcry came later and wouldn't immediately affect his work. Dr. Josef Mengele would be the most infamous, the "Doctor of Death," whose experiments at Auschwitz were among the most horrifying of the Nazi medical atrocities. Mengele especially prized twins for their research possibilities: in one typical series of experiments he would inject one twin with a deadly germ. Upon death, he would kill the surviving twin, and then compare the pair's organs at autopsy. Although Mengele would escape to South America after the war, twenty-three doctors would be tried at Nuremberg. While the trial became popularly known as "The Doctors' Trial," the U.S government focused on Hitler's personal physician and the star defendant in its title: *The United States v. Karl Brandt.*

Brandt was the son of a German policeman, born in 1904 in the region of Alsace. It was a beautiful, fertile area that Germany was forced to cede to France in the aftermath of World War I. The seizure of his homeland was the root of Brandt's fanaticism.

Brandt completed medical school in 1928, and joined the Nazi Party in 1932, heavily influenced by the party's promise to return Alsace to Germany. Brandt was also ambitious, and recognized the Nazi Party as the place to be for a man on the move. His opportunism was rewarded in 1933, when he was called on to treat Hitler's niece after an auto accident. Brandt was soon Hitler's number one medical authority.

Brandt also became the leading advocate of euthanasia for those people not perfect enough to contribute to the Third Reich. With Hitler's endorsement, Brandt headed Operation T-4, the program that killed children born with birth defects, malformities, or "idiocy." Brandt articulated the Nazi Party line when he argued that in a time of war and crisis, the state could not be expected to devote resources to the care of the handicapped. Soon enough, the category of "garbage children" was expanded to include Jews.

While Brandt's specialty was racial purification through euthanasia, he was also an enthusiastic advocate and participant in experimentation on human beings: Nazi doctors under Brandt's supervision dropped prisoners in icy water to see how long they would survive. Prisoners were locked in low-pressure barometric chambers until death. Battle-type wounds were painfully simulated and deliberately infected. Captives were forced to drink only seawater until dying to study the effects on lifeboat crews. The crime singled out as "perhaps the most utterly repulsive" by American Brigadier General Telford Taylor, the Nuremberg prosecutor, was the assembly of the Jewish skeleton collection. To confirm Nazi theories about the subhuman nature of the Jewish people, the doctors proposed to "induce" the deaths of as many Jews as possible, decapitate their corpses, and send their skulls to a lab for analysis. Eventually 115 people had their deaths "induced" in order to lend their skulls to the Nazi's bogus scientific pursuit.

The crimes of Brandt and the rest of the Nazi doctors would become well known during the Doctors' Trial, which took place from December 9, 1946, until August 19, 1947. Much less well-known than the Nazi experiments were the equally barbaric medical experiments performed by Japanese doctors during World War II. The Japanese experiments escaped notice largely because of a deal struck with the Americans, a deal personally approved by General Douglas MacArthur, the Supreme Commander of Allied Powers in Japan. In it, MacArthur agreed to give the Japanese scientists immunity from prosecution in exchange for the knowledge they had gained about biological and chemical warfare with their experiments. Like the Nazis, many of the Japanese test subjects were prisoners of war. The Japanese called their test subjects *maruta*—Japanese for "logs of wood." No one knows exactly how many of the *maruta* died at the hands of Japanese scientists, but even the Japanese admit that it was at least three thousand.

Their experiments were conducted mainly by a top secret Japanese military-medical detachment known as Unit 731 in occupied China. Their work included freezing limbs until they fell off, research done in anticipation of a land war in the frigid Soviet Union. The Japanese also experimented with mummifying victims alive with total dehydration, and with the replacing of every drop of a human's blood with the blood of a horse.

Unit 731 scientists even developed a starvation experiment of their own—it was conducted in response to the embarrassing revelation that many troops of the Imperial Army were suffering from malnutrition. The Japanese scientists wanted to find out what the limits of hunger were for troops in the field. In the experiment, two prisoners were made to continuously circle a course within a walled compound wearing forty-pound back-packs. The men were allowed to consume only small amounts of army biscuits and water. Both men were dead in two months.

After the war, unsullied by a war crimes trial, many of the Unit 731 scientists went on to become respected pillars of the Japanese scientific community. Dr. Kazu Tabei, who fed typhoid germs to prisoners by mixing them into milk, went on to become a professor of bacteriology at Kyoto University. Dr. Hisato Yoshimura, who froze captives to death, went on to become an adviser to the Japanese Antarctic Expedition and a consultant to the frozen food industry. Lieutenant Colonel Ryoichi Naito, whose unit had replaced a living human's blood with the blood of a horse, went on to found the Green Cross Corporation, an international pharmaceutical giant whose products include artificial blood.

Nuremberg was still in the future as Keys began his experiment. The Japanese medical atrocities would remain largely unknown. Keys' test subjects were volunteers, and, to the extent that he could, he informed them of the risks. When he did so, Keys was driven only by his own ethical standards, not because any international regulations or code forced him to.

CHAPTER FOUR

———◇———

CONTROL

HENRY SCHOLBERG stepped from the train station on November 19, 1944, into the coldest winter day he had ever known. He had arrived in Minneapolis, land of his forefathers. He sucked in his breath and tried to remember what he was supposed to do next.

A friendly cab driver offered refuge. "She's all warmed up for you," he said, getting out and slapping the hood with a mittened hand. The man smiled warmly. Henry bounded down the steps, and jumped into the snug cocoon of the taxi that smelled pleasantly of coffee and pipe tobacco. The driver shut Henry's door with a flourish and plopped down behind the steering wheel. He seemed to relish the cold.

"Where are we going today, son?"

"The University of Minnesota," said Henry. He fumbled through the brown envelope that held his CPS paperwork looking for more specific information.

"Whereabouts?" asked the driver. "That's a big campus, you know. Biggest in the country!"

Henry found the piece of paper he was looking for and read it twice. "The football stadium," he said, as much a question as a statement.

The driver laughed. "The football stadium? The final home game was last week you know—we beat Indiana somehow. I don't know about you, but I can't wait until the navy gives us Coach Bierman back."

"Yes—me too," said Henry. Although not a sports fan, Henry had spent four years at the University of Illinois, another Big Ten school, long enough to have heard of Minnesota's famous coach. He did not know that the coach had been uprooted by the war as well. "I hope he . . . comes back safe."

The driver roared with laughter at this. "Oh, I think he will. He's coaching a football team for the navy at a flight school in Iowa. Yeah, I think Coach Bierman will make it through the war without a scratch. So, are you sure you want to go to the stadium?"

Henry shook his head. "I guess . . . it sounds strange to me, too. I'm reporting to the Laboratory of Physiological Hygiene. I suppose it's in the stadium."

"Reporting," said the driver. "Reporting," he said again, still facing Henry. Henry watched as the man made the connection and his expression fell. Maybe he had read a newspaper article about the lab. The lab's use of COs was well known. Maybe he had seen the letters "CPS" on some piece of Henry's paperwork. In any case, Henry watched as he was transformed in the man's mind from a brave soldier home for Thanksgiving leave into a CO: a "conchie," a slacker, a coward. When the driver's grin had completely turned into a scowl, he turned around, threw the cab into gear, and drove them away from the station.

The rest of the drive through a quiet, Sunday morning Minneapolis was in silence.

As they drove down University Avenue, Memorial Stadium came into view, a massive brick horseshoe surrounding the white rectangle of the playing field. Henry saw countless empty rows of benches paralleling the field, each covered with an even layer of snow. The driver crossed a massive empty parking lot to the bottom of the U, to a huge gate that was obviously the stadium's main entrance. There wasn't another soul in sight.

"Is this . . . " said Henry. "Maybe this isn't the right place."

"It's the only football stadium we've got," said the driver without turning around.

Henry didn't relish the idea of being abandoned in that parking lot, but he had the distinct impression that the driver wasn't about to invite him home for lunch. He got out and pulled his small bag behind him. The driver took his fare from Henry without a word, and sped away.

Henry walked up to the entrance. A steel grate was drawn against the closed door, secured by a heavy black chain and padlock. Drawn by the arch, Henry's eyes traveled upward. Above the arch, on a massive stone tablet, idealized soldiers were carved in relief. An inscription read THIS STADIUM WAS ERECTED BY MEMBERS AND FRIENDS OF THE UNIVERSITY TO HONOR THE MEN AND WOMEN OF MINNESOTA WHO SERVED THEIR COUNTRY IN TIME OF WAR.

"Maybe this isn't the right place," Henry said again. His breath turned white, and floated away.

Henry walked the circumference of the stadium, feeling the cold Minnesota wind cut him with each gust. He had no doubt that a childhood in India had thinned his blood—no trace of his hearty Minnesota ancestors remained to brace him against the weather. He passed gates at regular intervals, each of them locked solidly in the same manner as the first. As he rounded the south arm of the U, he saw others like him, slightly confused young men keeping their heads down like veteran COs. He followed them to Gate 27, which he saw to his immense pleasure was labeled as the entrance to the Laboratory of Physiological Hygiene. With a numb hand, Henry pulled on the door and it opened. He went inside.

The space was unheated, but at least it was sheltered from the wind. When his eyes adjusted, Henry read a sign on the opposite wall.

Civilian Public Service
Unit 115
Sponsored by Brethren Service Committee
Headquarters Upstairs
Experimental Laboratory Downstairs

Someone who looked like he knew what he was doing came in behind him, and went upstairs. Henry followed.

Henry walked through a catacomb-like brick passageway. Mottled light from small, high windows and bare bulbs in cages showed the way. At regular intervals, the passageway would flare open into a room, revealing tables, treadmills, and alarming man-sized movable panels that appeared to be fitted with restraints. Finally, Henry reached a door that looked newer and had a fresher coat of paint than anything else he had passed. He stepped through the door into the room that would be his home for a year.

It was a long, warm, brightly lit space with two rows of cots neatly facing each other. A handful of other volunteers had already arrived, and were unpacking, shaking hands, and trying to look like they weren't nervous. There were no bunk beds, Henry was surprised to see—after a year in CPS, he had come to see bunk beds almost as an emblem of alternative service. The ceiling sloped upwards in a stair-stepped shape, mirroring the stadium seats over their heads. An empty footlocker stood open at the end of each cot, and government linens were stacked in perfect squares in the middle of each mattress. Although the room was not decorated in any way, and had no windows, there was something comfortable about it. Compared to the living conditions at the soil conservation camp in Lagro, Indiana, it was downright homey. Henry walked between the two rows of cots until he found an unclaimed bed that looked inviting.

To his left, a volunteer sat crosslegged on his bed with his eyes shut, loudly singing hymns. To his right, a volunteer unpacked photographs of his family. Something familiarly exotic in the photographs caught Henry's eye—there were palm trees and ancient temples in the background.

"I'm Henry Scholberg," he said to the man unpacking photos.

"Jay Garner," he said, extending his hand. "Pleased to meet you."

Henry was just about to ask about the setting of the photographs when a loud voice boomed from the entrance of the room.

"Is anyone hungry yet?" the newcomer said, arms raised. All conversation ceased as the rest of the volunteers turned to look at the new arrival. After a lengthy pause in the doorway, the man dropped his arms and strode dramatically down the center of the room, grinning broadly. Henry thought that the man smiled as if in response to applause heard only inside his head.

"What's the story with that mug?" Henry asked out loud as he walked by.

"His name is George Ebeling," said Garner. "We were in a Friends forestry camp together. He's an actor."

"Oh, I see," said Henry, because he could tell that Jay thought this explanation enough for the man's strange behavior. Henry continued unpacking. He noted with relief that Ebeling found a bed far from his, where he began loudly introducing himself to his openmouthed new neighbors. Henry was fighting back a sarcastic comment when a staff member in a lab coat appeared at the foot of his bed with a clipboard and a jar.

"Cedric Scholberg?" he asked.

He winced. "I go by Henry."

"I need a sample of your sperm," the man said.

Henry thought it over. "I think there's been a mistake," he said to the scientist. "I came here to get away from crazy people."

Before the flustered staff member could respond, another shouted from the middle of the room. "Please proceed downstairs to the laboratory," he said to the group. "You'll have time to unpack later on." Scholberg happily took the opportunity to escape the jar-wielding staffer by following the group out of the barracks and through the catacombs of the stadium. Their voices bounced excitedly off the brick walls of the stairwell as they descended. At the bottom of the stairs, above the door to the laboratory, was a sign with two biblical quotes: LET EVERY MAN PROVE HIS OWN WORK, followed by WHATSOEVER IS SET BEFORE YOU, EAT, ASKING NO QUESTION FOR CONSCIENCE SAKE. Below that sign, at the door of the laboratory, a doctor greeted them each stiffly with a hello and a handshake. He had short, dark, meticulously combed hair. His white lab coat was tailored to fit his robust, blocky frame. When Henry saw him, he had no doubt that it was Dr. Ancel Keys, and that he was the man in charge.

Keys knew that the appearance of the Laboratory of Physiological Hygiene did not live up to its grandiose name. Exposed pipes and conduit ran everywhere; only electrical panels adorned the concrete walls. The low ceilings looked like they could be a problem for some of the taller men when their turns came on the treadmills that were crammed into every corner. Keys was immensely proud of what he had accomplished beneath the football stadium and couldn't care less about appearances. Nevertheless, with the new group arriving, he couldn't help but see it through their eyes, and it looked a little drab. The setting had one advantage to Keys: sheer physical space. Dr. Keys had forty rooms at his disposal beneath the stadium, and despite their dungeon-like character, it was the only venue on campus where he would have enough room to house and test thirty-six volunteers. The next home football game wasn't until September 22, 1945, more than ten months away. Until then, Keys reigned over the largest structure at the University of Minnesota.

Keys greeted each man personally as he came through the door. They all looked healthy, the doctor was happy to see. They were a good-looking group as well, clean-cut and bright-eyed. Keys was consciously formal with each handshake. He was aware that at forty years old, he could be accused of being a bit young to be in charge of so much. Even so, as he watched these young men joke and shake hands with each other in the windowless lab, Keys felt like an old man.

When they had all arrived, Keys walked into the middle of the lab, and a hush fell over the room.

"Good morning," he said. He began the speech that he had spent the previous night rehearsing in front of Margaret. "We are here because of the problem of relief feeding in general, and particularly in the war devastated areas today. Accurate scientific data on the effects of starvation is almost completely lacking, and until it can be supplied, no really efficient program of relief can be planned or operated." Keys saw that he had calculated correctly in beginning the speech with the humanitarian goals of the study—the volunteers were rapt.

"At what levels of feeding calories, proteins, and vitamins is rehabilitation most rapid and most efficient? How long can we expect famine victims to be reduced in work capacity? What are the particular areas of human function most affected? The answers to these, and a host of more detailed technical questions, must be provided if the most effective use is to be made of any resources for relief, no matter how small or how large.

"Direct observations of famine victims in the field do not supply the answers because the necessary information on their pre-famine status is lacking and because field conditions are unsuitable for the collection of sufficiently exact information. It is fortunate that it was possible to establish this controlled project which bids fair, if not to yield all the answers, at least to greatly reduce the area of our ignorance on the questions of vital human interest.

"Human misery and want are qualities of life which properly bring an emotional response, but starvation is *quantitative* . . .

and must be met with quantitative answers. The service committees, the medical foundations, the University of Minnesota, and, not least, you, the volunteer subjects, have joined in a common effort to supply basic knowledge on how to achieve the highest food relief with fixed and obviously inadequate food resources. If our results allow an increase in efficiency of relief feeding by as little as five percent, we shall be able to reduce the sum of starvation suffering by an amount incalculably greater than would be possible with the same effort and expenditure on direct relief. And this gain is not limited to this year; it would extend to all time and all future food crises."

Keys let that hang in the air. It was exactly what the men had wanted to hear. He had omitted any reference in his speech to this group of pacifists about furthering the spread of Democracy and the American Way, just as he had downplayed the altruistic aspects of the study when selling it to the army. In fact, Keys believed in both justifications. What excited him the most, though, was the journey down an untraveled scientific road. No one had ever scientifically studied starvation, one of the most fundamental, common, and dangerous challenges faced by the human species. It was the career-making business of doing something for the first time, like drawing arterial blood at 20,000 feet. Keys kept that particular motivation to himself.

"Are you ready to begin?" he asked. A cheer erupted.

With that, his staff fell upon the volunteers, weighing and measuring them in every way that a man can be quantified. Weight was, of course, the signature datum for the duration of the study. At the outset, the men averaged 152.7 pounds. The heaviest among them, the Methodist L. Wesley Miller from Enid, Oklahoma, weighed 183.9 pounds. The lightest, little Bob Villwock, of the Evangelical Reformed Church in Toledo, Ohio, weighed only 136.4.

Calculating the amount of fat stored on each man's body was almost as crucial. Fat was the body's energy storage mechanism, an insurance policy taken out in plentiful times against future famines. Keys and the scientists were keenly interested in measuring how fat would deplete as the hungry body consumed itself. Body fat was measured by placing each subject on one end of a giant balance in the university swimming pool, and comparing the resulting weight to his weight on dry land. In scientific terms, they were measuring the *specific gravity* of the men. Because of the differing densities of muscle and fat, the difference in the two weights was directly related to the guinea pig's quantity of stored fat. During the control phase, body fat accounted for an average of about 14 percent of each man's weight, or about 21.6 pounds.

More exotic measurements included heart size, total blood volume, hearing, vision, and even sperm count—Scholberg's escape from that test proved to be temporary, as he and the rest of the volunteers took turns masturbating into wide-mouthed glass jars while Keys' technicians waited outside the bathroom door with cork stoppers.

The sperm analysis was emblematic of the thoroughness with which Keys planned to look at the men. The inquest began with a scientific question so general as to be almost philosophical: how does one of man's most fundamental drives affect another? In addition to closely tracking sexual dreams and thoughts in their mandatory journals and regular psychological screenings, the scientists devised a series of tests that analyzed sperm in every possible way. The ejaculate's volume was measured, as was its viscosity, clarity, and pH. The sperm count was carefully made, and motility was subjectively measured: estimates were made through a microscope as to the number of sperm making "active, purposeful, progressive movement through the liquid of the semen." The speed and the aggressiveness of the sperm were graded from 1 to 4. Finally, the sperm was placed in a refrigerator at 10°C and examined at four-hour intervals until all the aggressive, purposeful movement of the sperm had slowed to a stop. In 1944, all the analysis was laboriously manual, performed with pipettes, stirring sticks, and microscopes. The calculations were performed with slide rules, and the results were recorded long-hand in pencil on log sheets and added to a hill of data that would become a mountain in twelve months.

For each man, Keys had already constructed a weight-loss curve, a ski-slope-shaped graph that predicted each man's decreasing weight throughout the course of the starvation phase. Mathematically, the curve was a parabola, beginning at the far left at S1, the first day of the starvation phase, with the man's initial weight. The curve sloped downward across the twenty-four-week starvation phase to a point denoting a 25 percent weight loss. The curve was as prescriptive as it was predictive. Individual diets would be adjusted on a meal-by-meal basis—usually by tailoring the amount of potatoes—to keep each man on his curve. S1 was twelve weeks away.

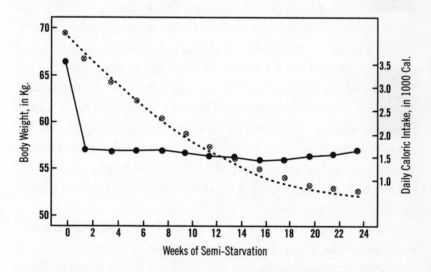

The Predictive Curve (from *The Biology of Human Starvation*).
The dotted line is weight loss, the solid line is caloric intake.

They were in C1, the first week of the twelve-week control period. Besides accumulating baseline data for each man, the goal of the control period was to determine each man's caloric "break even" point, the exact amount of food intake at which he would neither gain nor lose weight for a specific activity level. During this time, the men learned, their diet would be monitored and controlled to the last crumb, but it would not be deficient. A typical lunch served on January 25 consisted of fricasseed lamb with gravy, peas, and a carrot and raisin salad. For dinner a week later, the men ate roast beef with gravy, whipped potatoes, tomato salad, and ice cream for dessert. The three meals a day added up to about 3,200 calories. While the men were told that the diet was supposed to approximate normal American consumption, most admitted that they had never in their lives eaten so well.

Even during the control period, the cardinal rule of the study was this: the volunteers could only eat food provided by the lab. The meals were cooked and served at Shevlin Hall, on the opposite end of campus from the stadium. The kitchen at Shevlin had been completely given over to Keys for the duration of the experiment. A full-time cook, two assistants, and a dietician weighed each portion of food to the fraction of the ounce. Shevlin Hall was one of the oldest buildings on campus, built in the renaissance revival fashion in 1905. The men walked to their dining room through a two-story wood-paneled hall, complete with a massive stone fireplace and multicolored stained-glass windows. The cathedral-like setting helped establish the feeling that for the next twelve months, eating and food would be matters of almost sacramental importance.

Dr. Keys endeavored to keep each man busy for the duration of the experiment. He assigned each volunteer a job within the lab that was supposed to occupy about fifteen hours a week. Some men did general maintenance or laundry. Those with any kind of scientific background helped with lab work, tabulating data, or analyzing blood samples. A major block of each man's time was occupied by walking—each subject was required to walk twenty-two miles a week. The required treadmill time in the lab and the two to three miles a day covered in walking to and from Shevlin Hall did not count towards this total. All this activity was to stay constant through the starvation phase.

The men learned much about each other as they spent hours bound together by their tight living quarters and the constraints of the experiment. Everyone, it seemed, had an interesting story to tell. Henry Scholberg found out that Jasper "Jay" Garner, his barracks neighbor, had also spent his childhood in India and that his parents were Brethren missionaries. Jay had even gone to the same English-language school as Henry in Mussoorie, in the foothills of the Himalayas, where they had spent a year together as eight-year-olds. Jay told Henry how his family trekked into the darkest jungles to spread the word of God—at one point their Indian guides had the toddler Jay ford a stream with gourds tied around his arms, a primitive flotation device. George Ebeling, he of the dramatic entrance into the lab, was an accomplished actor and a member of the Hedgerow Theater Company in Pennsylvania. Harold Blickenstaff was the son of the Rev. L. C. Blickenstaff, one of the founding fathers of the CPS and director of CPS Camp Number 1 in Manistee, Michigan. The elder Blickenstaff had gone to prison for his pacifist beliefs during World War I, where he did time in Leavenworth alongside Eugene Debs, Socialist leader and five-time candidate for president.

During the well-fed control period, the men took pleasure in their long walks as they learned the campus and the surrounding city. They debated among themselves whether it was better to walk the entire twenty-two miles in a couple of long walks, or to spread it out evenly across the week. Henry Scholberg found that the twelve-mile round trip to the Ford Bridge was a satisfying long walk. For shorter jaunts, the Franklin Avenue Bridge was just three and a half miles away. There were plenty of other pleasing routes within the picturesque city to choose from. The campus occupied the east bank of the Mississippi River, Minneapolis's dominant natural feature. The university was directly across the river from downtown. Grain silos dotted the skyline, monuments to flour manufacturing, the city's major industry. Both General Mills and Pillsbury were headquartered in Minneapolis. Everywhere there was water. Besides the river, there were twenty-two natural lakes within the city limits. With complete freedom of motion in the beginning, the men had only their conscience to keep them out of the restaurants and bakeries of Minneapolis as they walked.

In addition to the endless testing, walking, and working, Keys scheduled twenty-five hours a week of instruction, classes in language, sociology, and political science. This was the "relief academy" he had promised the men, a training program for them to help the hungry directly at some unspecified future date, even as their bodies were yielding data for that same purpose. Some of the classes were taught by guest speakers invited by Keys, some by university faculty, and some even by test subjects with their own areas of expertise. Sam Legg volunteered to teach French, and his classes soon became favorites. By virtue of his expertise and his Princeton degree, Legg became the unofficial leader of the education program, a role he was happy to accept. Sam also had seniority within the CPS. He had been in since August 28, 1941, more than three months before Pearl Harbor. The median induction date for the men of the experiment was December 18, 1942. Only one man in the experiment had been in the CPS longer than Sam—Lester Glick, the experiment's only Mennonite, who had been inducted two months before Legg. Sam taught his French courses in a squash court. The underbelly of the stadium was studded with them along with handball courts and weight rooms. Basic French vocabulary ricocheted off the walls and the polished wood floor of the enclosed court as they learned. *Disputer:* to fight. *Aimer:* to love. *Manger:* to eat.

Conjugating French verbs and teaching helpful phrases for relief workers was a welcome distraction for Legg from his mother's increasingly frantic letters reporting his brother's latest misdeeds. Sam patiently explained in his responses that he couldn't come home to help her, he was absolutely committed to stay in Minnesota for a year.

One of Sam's students was Henry Scholberg, who soon outgrew the basic course Sam was teaching in the stadium. Henry enrolled in graduate level university courses in the language, and even joined the student French club, the Cercle Français. To his surprise, Henry was well-accepted by his fellow students, and not ostracized because of his status as a conscientious objector. He was even cast as Cléonte, the handsome boyfriend, in the club's production of Molière's *Le Bourgeois Gentilhomme*. Henry joked that it was a profound statement on the shortage of eligible young men on campus during wartime. He relished the classes and the rehearsals.

Henry wasn't the only guinea pig looking for stimulation outside the laboratory. Max Kampelman had written the NYU law school, asking if he could finish up what remained of his law degree with classes at the University of Minnesota. While he had passed the bar exam early before leaving New York, he still needed to complete his degree. The year on campus with free tuition seemed like the ideal opportunity. NYU agreed to accept the University of Minnesota credits.

Max was more worried about the University of Minnesota agreeing to the plan. The school was holding many of the law school's slots open for returning veterans. In addition, Max was from out of state, a part-time student, a conscientious objector, and not paying tuition. It would have been easy for the Minnesota law school to deny him a place. As Max would say years later, though, "Minnesotans are inclined to work things out." Everett Fraser, the dean of Minnesota's law school, approved Max's enrollment without comment.

Just as he was beginning his law classes early in the control phase, Max learned that he was scheduled to take something called the "Harvard Fitness Test" in the laboratory. It would be, he was told, the central measurement of each man's overall physical fitness throughout the experiment. Each man would take the test twice during the control period. Several already had taken it and reported on the grisly details to their rapt peers. Max found it hard to believe some of the reports, about running to complete exhaustion and collapsing on the racing treadmill, but the test had nonetheless become an object of almost mythological dread among the guinea pigs. Max was not immune. It was always administered in the mornings. Max could hardly sleep the night before, he was so worried. He nervously reported to the treadmill the next morning in track shorts and a T-shirt, where the scientists were waiting for him with clipboards and stopwatches.

"Do you know what we're about to do?" asked one with a clipboard.

"Let's hear it," said Max, trying to sound cavalier.

"You're going to walk for twenty minutes at first, at 3.5 miles per hour, at a 10 percent grade. After that, we're going to reduce the grade slightly, to 8.6 percent, and double the speed, to 7 miles per hour."

"How long do I do that?" asked Max.

"For five minutes or until you can't run anymore."

"How will you know when I can't run any more?" asked Max. A man stepped up from the shadows. Max hadn't seen him there; it was Dr. Keys.

"Max," he said somberly, "a test like this, a maximum capacity test, requires that you push yourself to the absolute limit, and continue until the last possible second of endurance. The validity of the test depends on it. This is one of the most important parts of our work here—this is one of the ways we will determine how much the capacity for work decreases among the hungry."

"So . . ." Max said. His question still hadn't been answered.

"You'll run until you collapse," said Keys.

"Very well," said Max. Now he realized why two men stood at the end of the treadmill. They were there to catch him. He stepped onto the treadmill, and the technician in charge flipped a switch to start the belt's motion.

Three and a half miles per hour was a brisk but not unbearable walking pace. Even so, Max was aware of a thin film of sweat that was starting to build on his forehead. His breath was quickening, and he found himself wondering when the twenty minutes would end. He didn't want to run out of gas before the run even started.

"Are you ready Max?" said the technician. Max nodded, trying to look confident while saving his breath. He heard a switch click into place.

The treadmill quickly doubled in speed. Max was able to keep up at first, but he soon felt his gait change from a disciplined, organized stride into a wild pounding. He lost track of time. He felt a stabbing pain in his side. He heard the words of Keys in his head, about pushing himself to the absolute limits of endurance, when finally his feet went out from under him. The two technicians were in place to catch him, but he fell slightly sideways, and his chin smashed onto one of the rails before they could stop his fall. Max bit his tongue painfully.

They carried the breathless, bleeding Max to a cot, where the main technician grabbed his wrist and began counting his pulse.

"How long did I last?" lisped Max, when he had regained his breath enough to speak. He tasted blood.

The technician didn't answer him, as he continued counting Max's pounding heart beats, and periodically wrote a number down. After recording three different pulse rates, the man pulled a slide rule from his shirt pocket, performed a calculation, and wrote a final number down next to Max's name: 44.

"How long did I last?" Max asked again.

"One hundred ninety-three seconds," said the man.

"Is that good?"

"Your score is forty-four—at the bottom of the 'average' category." He showed Max how the score was calculated, a complex formula that took into account the duration of the run and three different pulse rates during recovery. He walked away from Max to show the data to Dr. Keys, who was walking briskly out of the room.

Max thought it over. He barely scored "average" after two weeks of normal meals and miles of walking around campus, getting in shape. When he compared notes with the other men, he found that twelve men had gone the full five minutes, Henry Scholberg among them. Those twelve had a score in the "good" category. Bob Willoughby, a strapping Brethren farm boy from Harrisburg, Pennsylvania, was evaluated to be the fittest among them. No one had scored in the "superior" category. Seventeen men, like Max, were average. Three men were already in the "poor" category. Max contemplated what that mad run on the treadmill would feel like after six months of starvation.

All of the men intently followed the events of the war. The Minneapolis newspapers, the *Star Journal* in the morning and the *Tribune* in the afternoon, were the main sources of information, although little Bob Villwock's radio in the laundry room and newsreels in town were also occasionally informative. D-day had occurred on June 6, 1944, five months before the start of the experiment, and in general the Allied forces seemed to be steadily retaking Europe. There was a general feeling among the volunteers—and the rest of America—that Allied victory was within sight. That confidence was shattered on December 16, 1944, one month into the experiment, when the Germans launched a fierce, last-ditch counterattack in the snow-covered Ardennes. The German goals were to split the Allied line and retake Antwerp. History would know it as the Battle of the Bulge.

While the battle raged for the next twelve days, much of the news from the front was censored in the United States, especially in the early moments of the battle when the surprised American forces were reeling: "Allied military authorities directing the battle said it had been decided not to make public specific information now as to the exact places where the German columns were smashing through." Despite the censorship, there was no disguising the fact that something very serious was happening in the Ardennes. The first headline regarding the battle in the *Star Journal* read: GERMAN ATTACK TEARS HOLES IN 1ST ARMY LINES. Three days later, the headline read: NAZI PUSH CALLED WORST ALLIED SETBACK SINCE '42. If there was any doubt as to the gravity of the situation, the paper also announced that the Minnesota draft boards would be taking a close look at all men under twenty-six who had somehow managed to avoid the draft thus far. Daily lists of casualties from the area enumerated some of the spaces in the line that new draftees were needed to fill.

While the volunteers of the starvation experiment were pacifists, they felt no conflict in praying for an Allied victory. The men realized that it was America that gave them the opportunity to exercise their religious pacifism. They had no illusions that a fascist government would give them that same chance. Many of the men had friends and family in the fight. Jay Garner's brother had defied his father, the Brethren missionary, by joining the navy. Charles Smith, a Baptist volunteer from Merchantville, New Jersey, had a brother in the army. While unable to fight in the war themselves, the volunteers had no problem identifying the good guys and the bad guys in the current struggle.

Those feelings were confirmed when news of the massacre at Malmedy, Belgium, reached Minneapolis. Seventy-one unarmed American POWs were machine-gunned down by officers of the SS in a snow-covered clearing. It was one of the worst atrocities committed against American troops during the war. The Battle of the Bulge raged until December 26. More than a million soldiers were in the fight. The 81,000 American casualties were the heaviest of any battle of the war.

The patriotic inclinations of the volunteers would have hardened further had they known about another landmark of the war that took place on January 27, 1945. As the control phase of the experiment neared its end, four Russian cavalrymen came upon a fenced camp in Auschwitz-Birkenau, Poland. At first they thought it abandoned. When they moved closer, they saw men moving through the snow like ghosts, men they described as "living skeletons." The retreating Nazis had tried unsuccessfully to destroy any evidence of the crimes they had committed there, at the headquarters of Dr. Mengele. It was impossible to erase every trace of crimes on that scale. In one room, the dumbstruck Russian soldiers found 14,000 pounds of human hair.

Like most Americans, the volunteers remained clueless about the Holocaust for most of the war. Some of this was due to an initial disbelief about the scope of the tragedy. Americans couldn't believe that a Western, civilized nation like Germany could perpetrate such crimes. Anti-Semitism was surely also a component of the early silence, as was the American government's longstanding fear that publicizing Hitler's crimes against the Jews would somehow distract Americans from military missions viewed as more critical. The American press's tendency to downplay achievements of the Red Army might also have been a factor in the lack of news about the liberation of Auschwitz. As the war lurched to a close all the Allied armies across Europe began to stumble across camps with living skeletons, and Americans began to comprehend the scope of the tragedy. When the twelve-week control phase ended on February 11, 1945, however, it would still be many months before Auschwitz was a household name.

Most of the men found themselves in good spirits after the first twelve weeks. On the "complaint inventory," one of the never-ending psychological tests they took, the most common complaint at the end of the control period was a "yes" in answer to the question "Do you find yourself often sleepy and/or tired during the day?" Forty-one percent of the men were so afflicted. When asked, "Does 'guinea pig' life seem to be a strain for you much of the time?" every one of the volunteers answered "no." They had, on average, already lost 1.76 pounds each. The caloric "break even point" at the end of the control period was on average 3,210 calories per day. On February 11, the men all knew that they were on the eve of sacrifice, discomfort, and even danger. At the end of C12, most were ready to begin the challenge. No one more so than Dr. Ancel Keys.

Sam Legg walked the dark, frozen campus alone, finishing up his twenty-two miles for the week. He knew that it would be his last such walk around campus with a relatively full stomach. It had snowed all day, and the wind that cut through the campus seemed to have blown directly from the North Pole. None of the old snow had melted. It was pushed aside by the plows each morning into giant, dirty mountains. The next day, Lincoln's Birthday, the starvation phase began. Rehabilitation wouldn't start until July 29. The snowdrifts and the bitter wind made that summer date seem impossibly far away. Legg knew that he was considered a leader of the group, confident and capable. So he had to keep his fears to himself. As he crossed the campus alone, marking his final mile, he wondered if he was strong enough.

CHAPTER FIVE

---◂◦▸---

CRUCIFYING THE FLESH

THE END OF THE WAR was in sight when the starvation phase began in Minnesota, on February 12. In fact, one day before, on February 11, 1945, Churchill, Stalin, and Roosevelt completed their conference in Yalta, where the "Big Three" had decided in advance what a postwar Europe should look like. Dr. Keys wanted each man's weight to slope downward over time, tracing the course of that predictive parabola. The decrease in calories would be more abrupt. Keys wanted the change to be sudden and shocking to the body, "as was the case during the 1941–42 siege of Leningrad." The group shifted overnight from the three relatively generous meals of the control period to only two Spartan meals per day, a breakfast at 8:30 AM and supper at 5:00 PM. The two meals supplied an average of 1,570 calories per day, roughly half that of the previous three months. Three menus were prepared for the men in rotation. All the while, the men maintained a constant activity level, attending classes, doing their assigned jobs, and walking twenty-two miles every week.

The meals were designed to approximate the food available in European famine areas, with a heavy emphasis on potatoes, cabbage, and whole wheat bread. Meat was provided in quantities so small that most of the men would swear in later years that none was included at all. Water, black coffee, chewing gum, and cigarettes were allowed in unlimited quantities. One of the three dinners included the following:

SUPPER #2

185 grams of bean-and-pea soup (made with
5 grams dried peas, 16 grams dried beans,
and 15 grams fresh ham)

255 grams macaroni and cheese (made with
130 grams wet macaroni, 12 grams lard, 108
grams skim milk, 2 grams flour, and 35 grams
American cheese)

40 grams rutabagas

100 grams steamed potatoes

100 grams lettuce salad (80 grams lettuce, 10
grams vinegar, 10 grams sugar)

The relatively bulky 255 grams of macaroni made that particular meal an anticipated favorite among the volunteers. The wet macaroni served was roughly the amount required to fill a coffee mug about three-quarters full.

Keys tracked only the vitamins A, thiamine, niacin, D, and C in the diets. The starvation diets contained adequate supplies of each, which was important, since Keys wanted to study the effects of starvation, not the effects of any specific vitamin deficiency. In 1945, the whole concept of vitamins was still new. The term *vitamin* had been coined in 1911 by Polish chemist Kasimir Funk, who thought the substances were "life's amines." A friend and colleague of Keys' at Cambridge, Dr. Albert Szent-Gyorgi, had won the 1937 Nobel Prize in Medicine for isolating and synthesizing vitamin C, or ascorbic acid, just seven years before the start of the starvation experiment. He was so proud of his discovery that he once showed Keys a test tube full of vitamin C crystals that he carried around in his vest pocket.

With few exceptions, the men were able to find humor in their hunger and decreasing size in the first few weeks. The study's lone Mennonite, Lester Glick, wrote in his diary on March 16, after the first month of starvation, "Wow! My clothes look sloppy! My belt buckle is in the last notch—a decrease of three notches since the starvation began." Other men complained, "the time between meals has now become a burden." All in all, most of the men were still buoyed by their noble motivations, and spirits remained high. Sooner than anyone expected, however, hunger began calling out the weak among them.

Franklin Watkins, Subject Number 234, walked quietly into the dark passageway. The cold air held that combination of smells peculiar to the stadium, a blending of medicinal alcohol from the lab and burnt popcorn from the previous football season. The brick walls and concrete floor were covered in a film of slimy condensation. It was late, and Watkins could hear the raspy snores of the other volunteers behind him as he sneaked away from the barracks. That sound was soon drowned out by the pounding of his heart in his ears and the growling of his stomach. There was a secret chamber somewhere in the stadium, he knew, a place where he could eat all he wanted without consequence or supervision. He was determined to find it.

He stumbled through the catacombs of the stadium, down stairways and through tunnels, until he saw the heavy, bolted door at the end of a blind passageway. It was a steel hatch, the kind you might find on a ship, set directly into a brick wall. The small red DO NOT ENTER sign seemed redundant on the forbidding door. Watkins spun the wheel mounted in its center. He heard an oily click as the tumblers of the lock fell into place. He pushed, and the heavy but precisely balanced door glided open.

Watkins stepped through. It was even darker inside. Soon enough, his eyes adjusted to the darkness, and he knew he had succeeded: he had found Dr. Keys' secret laboratory. There were old, withered people huddled in the corners, muttering nonsense in the dark. Younger lunatics wandered aimlessly through the room, bumping wordlessly into each other, the walls, and him. There was no telling what vital substances these men were being deprived of in the name of science. Maybe the scientists had forgotten about them in this remote corner of the stadium, as the starvation experiment occupied all their attention. The captives all seemed emaciated, weak, skeletal. Watkins barely felt an impact when one of them brushed against him, and continued on his way. He stepped deeper into the room.

He saw the man he was looking for huddled in a corner by himself. He was older and even smaller than the rest. In his weakness, he had been abandoned by the group, left to fend for himself. Watkins knelt to look at him directly. No fear or recognition registered in the old man's cloudy eyes. Sure now that he wouldn't resist, Watkins picked up the old man's arm and held it in front of him. The limb was light, as unsubstantial as a bird's wing. The old man calmly watched as Watkins put the wrinkled, gray arm into his mouth. Watkins took a gigantic bite. The old man began moaning loudly. Watkins feasted on the man's arm more urgently, though his victim was too weak to even attempt self-defense. Watkins had to eat fast, because Dr. Keys would be along to stop him soon enough. The skin was salty, dry, and tough, but the flesh inside was tender and juicy, like good pie or rare steak. The rest of the lunatics continued walking obliviously in circles. Blood ran down Watkins' chin as the old man wailed.

When Watkins snapped awake from the nightmare, he realized that the mournful wailing was coming from him. He sat erect in bed, catching his breath, scanning the dark room to see if his nightmare had disturbed anyone's sleep other than his own. Watkins was relieved that he was not cannibalizing a senile old man, but distressed to realize that he seemed to be losing his mind. Quitting was out of the question. One of the reasons he volunteered for the experiment was to disprove the notion that COs were weak or gutless; quitting would confirm that he was both, to the world and to himself. Cheating was slightly less abhorrent. Watkins felt guilty even about the meat he had consumed in the dream. But he had to make the nightmares stop. Illicit food seemed to be his only hope.

Watkins was the twenty-four-year-old son of a wealthy Pittsburgh family. He was a talented organist and fluent in German. He taught the language to would-be relief workers in a squash court adjacent to Sam Legg's under the stadium. Unlike many of the volunteers, the farm boys and the missionaries' sons, Watkins had never known real deprivation. He grew up having rich meals brought to him by servants. But it wasn't just the lack of food that made him come unhinged in Minneapolis, it was the regimentation. Keys wanted to know about every step he took, every thought he had, every dream. He tracked each morsel of food Watkins ate from before it was cooked until it was metabolized into a few ergs of energy as he panted on the treadmill. Watkins could feel the equation change on the first day of starvation, when the energy going out became greater than the food going in. He felt his body turn inward to consume itself. That's when he began dreaming of cannibalism.

In response, he began to cheat extravagantly. He gulped down sundaes and malted milks in town, as many as he could stomach. He ate two raw rutabagas stolen from the kitchen in Shevlin Hall. Still, the nightmares haunted him, every night.

Watkins' weight veered sharply from the predictive curve. Keys questioned him, and Watkins tearfully confessed to the cheating and vowed to do better, surrendering his checkbook and his cash. He also confessed to the scientist about his dreams of eating lunatics and old people.

While Watkins' dreams of cannibalism were disturbing, they were not altogether surprising to Keys. Cannibalism had always been linked to famine. While psychologists couldn't write a precise mathematical formula relating the severity of a famine to the number of cannibals it would generate, it was clear that at some point hunger would drive people to violate this most fundamental taboo, whether in Leningrad or the Old Testament. Second Kings 6:26–29 described such a famine: "Give thy son, that we may eat him today, and we will eat my son tomorrow. So we boiled my son, and did eat him." Keys noted with some interest in his historical survey on the subject that Asian peoples seemed somehow more resistant to the temptations of cannibalism. He theorized that perhaps the reasons were religious: "in the Orient the concept of the complete dissociation of body and soul is less fixed than in the Western world."

Despite surrendering his money, Watkins' descent continued, as he shoplifted what he could no longer buy. At meals and in the barracks, he began openly challenging the value of the experiment. "What are we really accomplishing here? What are we doing here? What kind of science is this?" He sought out those men who seemed to be suffering the most and tried to get them to quit with him in some kind of general strike. The other volunteers began avoiding him, heightening his isolation and depression.

When Watkins' aberrant weight loss clearly indicated a relapse, Keys again confronted him in his office in the stadium. "We know you're still cheating," he said. He stated it as scientific fact, not an accusation. He had no desire to hear the young man's excuses or lies. "I'm afraid we are going to have to restrict you to the stadium. You can no longer leave the laboratory alone."

Watkins began sobbing violently. "I'm a failure!" he screamed at Keys, who sat across from him coolly taking notes on his reaction. "I'm not good enough to be here!" Suddenly Watkins stood, tears still running down his face. "I'm going to kill myself!" he shouted at Keys between sobs. He pointed a shaky finger at the scientist. "I'm going to kill you!"

Keys sighed, put his pencil down, and rubbed his eyes. The stocky Keys, who had beaten a colleague to the ground atop a Chilean peak, was not afraid of Franklin Watkins. He was just disappointed, and profoundly irritated, to lose a man so soon. When the cheating began, he had hoped to keep the man in the experiment, but the violent threats made that impossible now. All that data lost. He picked up his telephone, and had Franklin Watkins taken to the psychiatric ward of the university hospital.

Within a few days of normal meals, Watkins showed no sign of psychosis and was released.

Keys was not sympathetic to Watkins in his summary of the incident. After all, the man was just a few weeks into the experiment when he began to buckle. Complete mental collapse came even before the halfway point. For all of Keys' stated goals about helping the helpless in Europe, he felt little compassion for the weak living inside his laboratory. He speculated that many clinicians would classify Watkins as "psychopathic." Additionally, he wrote that "the subject is a bisexual with poor personality integration and weak self control." Keys based his diagnosis of bisexuality only on the MMPI results and on Watkins' earlier admission that he had once had a "beautiful friendship" with a man years before.

For most of the test subjects, physical weakness and fatigue were the most noticeable effects of hunger during the first half of the experiment. The weakness manifested itself in a variety of ways. Henry Scholberg was one of the only volunteers to attempt dating while in Minneapolis. His companion one night near S12, a laboratory employee named Doris Fredson, was so diminutive that

she went by the nickname "Tini." In the lobby of the movie theater, Henry stared longingly at the popcorn as they walked by the
concession stand. Inside, Henry found himself unable to concentrate on the film, *To Have and Have Not,* except for a scene early
on where Humphrey Bogart was eating his dinner in a bar—
Henry stared as he put away each bite. Even the sultry Lauren
Bacall failed to interest him as much as Bogie's supper. As Henry
and Tini walked back to the stadium across the darkened campus, Henry warned her about his weakened state. "Tini," he said,
"if we're attacked, you should run like hell. I won't be able to
defend you." He failed to get a kiss good night.

Jay Garner, Henry Scholberg's classmate in India, ventured
from the lab that same week to visit Dayton's department store in
downtown Minneapolis. He looked forward to completing a
major part of his twenty-two-mile walk for the week, as well as
some enjoyable window-shopping. His journey came to a halt
when he became trapped in the store's revolving door—he no
longer had the strength to push it around. Garner waited embar-
rassed inside the door until a better-fed patron was able to push
the door and liberate him.

Keys was monitoring the decrease in physical strength among
the men with much interest. How starvation affected the capacity
for work was one of the major quests of the study. Strength, speed,
coordination, and endurance were all measured with the usual
thoroughness; of those four traits, strength showed the greatest
deterioration. During the first twelve weeks of starvation, the men
showed on average a 21 percent reduction in strength, as measured by the amount they could heft with the back lift dynamometer, a calibrated device that measured the maximum amount lifted
by each man. As the starvation phase neared its halfway point,
Keys heard that the character of the collapse during the dreaded
Harvard Fitness Test had changed. He decided to see for himself.

The test would be run in the morning, as always. During the
control phase, each man had taken the test twice, to obtain an

average score for each guinea pig. Because of the severe physical drain of the test, and because of the dread the men had attached to it, Keys had decided that the test would only be given twice for each man in the starvation phase—once at about the halfway point and once near the end. The test subject arrived in his track shorts and tennis shoes and did his best to look stoic as the technicians prepared to administer the test. Keys looked at the file. His name was Sam Legg.

By the numbers, he was a typical guinea pig in almost every way. He was 5 feet 10 inches tall, within an inch of the group's mean height. During the control phase, he had weighed 142.34 pounds, again very close to the average. His weight loss, twenty-six pounds or about 18 percent, had also been normal. Keys was glad that he had chosen such a representative subject to observe.

"Are you ready?" the technicians asked him. Legg nodded. They started the treadmill at 3.5 miles per hour. The rollers squeaked and Legg's rubber soles began to rhythmically thump the belt for the test's twenty-minute walk. Keys watched closely. By the end of twenty minutes, the subject was breathing heavily. During the control phase, they had told the men that they would run them for five minutes or until they couldn't run anymore. Now the qualifier was unnecessary—none of the men were getting anywhere close to five minutes.

"Ready to speed up?" asked the technician. Legg nodded. He had a strange look on his face, one that Keys' hadn't expected, and couldn't at first identify. He didn't look frightened, Keys observed, but he didn't look defiant either. The man was about to run until he collapsed from exhaustion, thought Keys, and there was no way to be enthusiastic about that, no matter how much good you might be doing for humanity.

The treadmill came up to speed. For a short while, Legg managed to keep up. Then his weakened state made itself apparent. In the control phase, the collapse had been foreshadowed by pounding feet, swaying, and a general loss of ground. Now, Keys could see a definite difference. Legg was just unable to keep up the pace, and was falling farther and farther behind. The result was a gradual lean forward, until it seemed he would fall flat on his face.

Collapse came at 106 seconds. The technicians, their task made easier with practice and with the reduced weights of the volunteers, caught him before his face hit the treadmill. They sat him on a bench and took his pulse rates and calculated his score while Keys watched.

A 32, down from a 72 in the control phase. From high in the "average" category to solidly in the "poor." Over all, a 55 percent decrease in fitness, which again put Legg solidly in the middle of the crowd. He was experiencing completely typical physical deterioration.

Keys watched the young man as the scientists completed taking his pulse rates and blood pressure. He looked for some sign of anger or depression about the dreadful test. Maybe even a sign of relief that at least he wouldn't have to do it again for a few weeks. Keys saw no sign of any of those. The look on Legg's face was exactly the same as when he had climbed on board the treadmill. It was an expression of profound resignation. Keys wrote in his notes on the changing nature of the collapse: "The picture is one of pure muscular weakness."

As Keys had foreseen when he designed the starvation study, the world's food situation continued to deteriorate throughout the course of the experiment. Continental Europe was especially hard hit. In addition to being the area under fire the longest (since the Nazi invasion of Poland in 1939), the region was dependent on food imports even in the best of times. Naval warfare brought the shipping of foodstuffs to a halt and almost completely stopped the fishing industry, another important source of animal protein on the continent. In an era when agriculture was still unmechanized and laborious, the war had decimated the workforce available to tend crops and care for livestock. Aggravating all of this was a stretch of severe winters and crop failures in Europe that predated and continued through the war. While some countries, like the United States, were still producing surpluses of grain and other commodities until late in the war, the war at sea and the destruction of railroads across Europe made it impossible to get American food into the hands of the hungry.

The idea that food would be a central issue in the world's postwar recovery received almost daily reinforcement in the newspapers that the Minneapolis test subjects pored over. A headline in the *Minneapolis Star Journal* on a Helen Kirkpatrick article datelined Paris, on February 26, 1945, read FRENCH FOOD CRISIS GROWS MORE CRITICAL. She described a mass demonstration of forty thousand Parisians that nearly developed into a full-blown food riot. She wrote that "France's four years of privation are beginning to show their effects in mounting tubercular deaths, in infant mortality, and in the rise of pernicious pneumonia."

An April 4 headline read ENOUGH FOOD DOESN'T EXIST. The article described the challenge of feeding civilians at home and starving people abroad. General Ralph Olmstead of the War Food Administration explained that after filling military requirements, there just wasn't enough food to go around. Nearing victory had ironically made the food problem worse. "Supply lines are longer, thousands of prisoners being taken must be fed and civilian relief needs increase as new areas are liberated."

Clare Boothe Luce's dispatch from Rome on April 11 was titled "Food Is Key to Politics in Italy." An Italian official she quoted succinctly made the same argument Keys had made in justifying the starvation experiment to military authorities the previous year. The Italian said they wanted the chance to bring their country "back again into the column of peaceful democratic nations. But this we cannot do while the Italian people face starvation and with it the threat of political chaos."

Another article from Helen Kirkpatrick on April 12 was titled

STARVATION RIDDEN HOLLAND A GROWING ALLIED PROBLEM. She explained that the death rate had risen 300 percent in Holland since the New Year, and that people were dropping dead in the street from starvation.

Not all food problems the men read about were overseas. The daily ads for Minneapolis grocery stores that taunted the hungry volunteers were divided into "points" sections and "no points" sections, signifying which foodstuffs were rationed and which were not. On March 15, 1945, for example, the A&P advertised leg of lamb at 35 cents and 7 points per pound; a fourteen-ounce jar of pig's feet was only 20 cents and no points. It was an indication that even with the end of the war supposedly in sight, rationing was still in full force in the United States, as the Office of Price Administration and the War Food Administration attempted to regulate growing shortages and stifle inflation. The *Minneapolis Star Journal* did a four-part series on the domestic food shortage just as the starvation phase began its sixth week.

Rationing had been in effect in the United States since shortly after the Japanese attack on Pearl Harbor in December 1941. Food was not the first commodity rationed—tires were, as Japan's rapid advance across the jungles of South Asia threatened America's rubber supply. Food rationing soon followed. Shortages were caused both by the direct effects of combat on agriculture and shipping around the world and by the huge nutritional demands of the military. Rationing, shortages, and hoarding would mark the duration of the war.

It was the first time the United States government had ever had to ration food to civilians, given its enormous resources and peaceful shores. In World War I, the government had exercised some limited control over food production, but had carefully avoided rationing to civilians. Instead, the government encouraged Americans to enjoy voluntarily one "meatless" and one "wheatless" meal per day. That war ended for the Yanks in eighteen months, long before any large-scale shortages could develop on American soil.

That request for belt-tightening would become a requirement in the Second World War. Leaders recognized early on that the United States would bear the burden for feeding the world as the war raged on. Without rationing and price controls, the U.S. government feared that supplies would dwindle, prices would skyrocket, and food would become available only to the rich. At best such conditions would undermine general support for the war effort. At worst food shortages and hunger might lead to unrest, rioting, or even more serious upheaval. Recognizing that domestic tranquility required an adequately fed populace, President Roosevelt moved early to implement government controls, forming the Office of Price Administration even before Pearl Harbor, in April 1941. Business interests and conservative economists were certain that it was just another attempt by the liberal Roosevelt to quash free enterprise, but most Americans seemed to recognize that despite its inconveniences, rationing was a program designed to protect them from profiteers and hoarders.

In May 1942, sugar became the first foodstuff rationed to civilians in American history. It would also be the last for which controls were lifted as sugar rationing would last until 1947. Americans throughout the war were allotted on average 24 pounds of sugar per year, approximately half of their prewar consumption. An extra allotment of 10 to 20 pounds could be obtained for use in canning and preserving food, an activity the government strongly encouraged. It was perhaps the shortage of sugar that Americans felt most acutely during the war. A July 1945 survey asked Americans to make a hypothetical choice between 25 pounds of sugar, 15 gallons of gasoline, 5 pounds of butter, or 5 pounds of steak. Sugar was the runaway winner of the poll. Sugar was rationed by its own special stamps, which were exchanged, along with money, for the product.

Coffee rationing began in November 1942. Canned goods joined the list on March 1, 1943; meat on March 29. Meat and canned goods were rationed by a more complicated system than sugar. Every American citizen was issued two booklets of ration stamps per month: one red with six stamps and one blue with five stamps. America's schoolteachers were asked to volunteer their time to issue the booklets. The rationing system, like the Selective Service System, made itself conspicuously democratic, with a strong emphasis on volunteers and local boards.

Red stamps were for meats, fats, and dairy. Blue stamps were for canned goods. Each stamp was worth ten points. "Change" was given with red and blue tokens. The point value of any particular food item varied over time and geographically, depending on local availability. The OPA relied on a volunteer board of 2,500 housewives across the country to keep food diaries, with which the point values of items were reevaluated every month. Margarine consumption soared with the rationing of butter. The nation's powerful dairy lobby, fearful that over the course of a long war American consumers might find the two products indistinguishable, insisted that a punitive federal tax be levied on margarine dyed yellow.

Rosie the Riveter, with her work shirt, flexed arm, and determined gaze, was an image used by the United States government to encourage wives and mothers to go into the workplace, filling those gaps in America's assembly lines created by men going to war. Though millions of wives and mothers had followed Rosie's example, it was still generally their task to take all the family's ration stamps, budget, and local availabilities into account to come up with a menu. It was a complicated job—just because you had the stamps and the money did not mean that a particular product would actually be available in any local groceries. The government helped by encouraging the use of alternative sweeteners, like corn syrup and molasses, which were not rationed. Similarly, homemakers were encouraged to try out the point-free "variety meats," the OPA's euphemistic term for organs. Patriotic Americans tried to acquire a taste for beef kidney pie, boiled tongue, and stuffed beef heart.

The war affected American diets in another fundamental way. Prepared and canned foods were rationed to the public because they were needed in huge quantities to ship overseas, for soldiers, persons in liberated areas, and prisoners. The OPA strongly encouraged Americans to grow "victory gardens" to reduce their consumption of canned foods. Americans responded in force. By 1943, three-fifths of the population were growing some of their own food, producing an astonishing 40 percent of the vegetables consumed in American homes. This bonanza of fresh vegetables was one nutritional side effect of the war of which Ancel Keys would have wholeheartedly approved.

On April 12, 1945, all the headlines about rationing and milk shortages were pushed to the back of the paper: Franklin Delano Roosevelt had died. The average twenty-five-year-old volunteer in the experiment had been a thirteen-year-old boy when FDR was first elected. To lose him when the end of the war was in sight seemed a terrible injustice.

Four days later, Ancel Keys called a meeting of the unit.

They filed nervously into the room. Keys was at the center, flanked by his colleagues Josef Brozek and Henry Longstreet Taylor. The guinea pigs knew it had to be something major. Keys had not called for a formal group meeting since he introduced himself on their first day. They had never been assembled in front of the entire senior staff in this way. Keys' somber look did nothing to alleviate their anxiety.

Keys stared at each man as he filed in, trying to discern who would be the next to crack. The men had been in the starvation phase for nine weeks. He thought that they looked gaunt, but not yet emaciated or sickly. Brozek nodded when the last guinea pig had filed in. Keys got quickly to the point.

"There has been cheating," he said. The guinea pigs were visibly shocked by the pronouncement. Like Keys, they had not expected someone to buckle so quickly. He continued. "Obviously, all data from that individual is now invalid, and his time here has been a waste. I must assume that the temptation to cheat has become too powerful. In light of this, there will be no more leaving the laboratory unaccompanied. We will implement a 'buddy system.' If you need to go outside these walls from now on, you must take someone from the lab with you."

The men began mumbling among themselves. Keys anticipated some of the questions in the crowd.

"There will be no exceptions for university classes, religious services, dating, or anything else. I realize this complicates matters greatly for some of you, but such are the necessities of experiment. I thank you all." As Keys left, the men noticed for the first time that Franklin Watkins had not made the meeting.

Keys was right—the buddy system did complicate matters. Now whenever Max Kampelman or anyone else went to class, he had to talk someone into sitting through a law lecture with him. What little dating had survived into the tenth week of starvation was now over.

Three days later, on April 19, 1945, Keys called another meeting and confirmed the rumors: Franklin Watkins was the cheater and had been released from the experiment. They were down to thirty-five men.

Two close friends in the experiment took the news about Watkins hard. They were James Plaugher and Bob Willoughby. The two men had much in common. While Willoughby had been evaluated as the "fittest" of the group during the control phase, based on the Harvard Fitness Test, James Plaugher had been judged the strongest, based on a test using a back-lift dynamometer. Plaugher was among the biggest men in the experiment, at 6 feet 3 inches and 182 pounds during the control phase. In a barracks filled with intellectuals and artists, Willoughby and Plaugher were jocks.

Willoughby had been a varsity basketball player at Elizabeth-town College, a Brethren school in Lancaster County, Pennsylvania. His athleticism was honed at CPS Camp 134, in Belden, California, where he had spent his days hiking up and down the steep canyons of Plumas County, surveying the forests and turning his legs into rock hard rods of muscle. Besides being the fittest man in the laboratory, Willoughby had been in the CPS the least amount of time. When the experiment began, Willoughby had been in only eight months.

So both Willoughby and Plaugher were more athletic than the average guinea pig in the lab, and both were more apt to discuss the upcoming football season than the next performance by the university's Shakespeare company. Their similarities might have made them friends anyway. The fact that they both came under a common cloud of suspicion drove them closer. Keys was convinced that both men were cheating.

Both Willoughby and Plaugher had had trouble losing weight almost from the beginning. By S12, Plaugher's weight had stalled out at 156 pounds. Willoughby was stuck at 139 pounds. The average weight at S12 was 125 pounds. This despite the fact that both Plaugher and Willoughby saw their diets slashed to the lowest level. While the average diet in starvation was 1,570 calories per day, Plaugher was subsisting on 1,200 calories a day and Willoughby on 1,100 at S12, as their weights stubbornly remained above their predictive curves. After the truth about Watkins came out, they started receiving increasingly pointed questions from the staff about cheating.

In one of these interviews, after much coaxing, Plaugher nervously confessed that he had in fact cheated on an infinitesimal scale: he had stolen a crust of bread from the kitchen early in the starvation phase. Willoughby maintained that he had not cheated at all. In any case, a single crust of bread would not explain the aberrant weight loss seen in both men.

The staff interpreted the quietness of the men in their interviews as evasiveness. Willoughby and Plaugher were both naturally reticent, even in their diaries, which contained far fewer entries than average. This frustrated Keys, who was used to the sometimes extravagant self-examinations given by the other, more articulate volunteers. The scientists, unable to confirm more cheating from Plaugher or any cheating at all from Willoughby, slashed their diets further in an attempt to bring their weights down to their predictive curves. Soon both men would be consuming less than 1,000 calories a day at Shevlin Hall.

In their nervousness and misery, Plaugher and Willoughby took advantage of a lab rule that allowed unlimited gum chewing. They began spending all their money on the stuff, chewing as much as forty packs a day. Their mouths hurt from chewing so much gum, and both men exhausted their limited finances on it. Plaugher chewed up and spit out so much that he measured his gum consumption with a beer mug. As their spirits sank and their gum chewing soared, the psychologists began watching both of the big men carefully.

In the first weeks of starvation, many of the men still had the energy and the motivation to avail themselves of the numerous artistic activities going on around campus. The options were refreshing for educated men who had spent years in forestry camps and remote mental hospitals. A group of four including Sam Legg, Marshall Sutton, Carlyle Frederick, and Bob Willoughby heard a string quartet in St. Paul on February 16. George Ebeling, he of the Hedgerow Theater, performed in a student production of George Bernard Shaw's *Candida* that same week. There were concerts, plays, musicals, and lectures constantly, proving Keys' assertion that his men had a higher than average interest in "cultural activities."

While by law all men came to the CPS for religious reasons, and while most of the men attended church through at least the first weeks of the starvation phase, religious differences rarely came up in barracks conversation. In general, the men were not even aware of the different denominations of their peers, although Max Kampelman did at first field a few curious questions from those men who had never before known a Jew. In later years, many of the men would share the common, incorrect assumption that the Historic Peace Churches supplied the majority of the guinea pigs. The men had so much in common as pacifists that they seemed to accept each other's different faiths without questions or friction. The hardships of the experiment soon erased whatever dim sectarian lines may have existed. While the Civilian Public Service no doubt had its share of fundamentalist zealots from all creeds, none had apparently made it to CPS Camp 115 under Memorial Stadium.

The death camp at Buchenwald, Germany, was liberated by American troops under General Eisenhower on April 11, eight weeks after the starvation phase began in Minnesota. The news didn't reach Minneapolis until days later. An April 23 *Star Journal* headline read BUCHENWALD CAMP ATROCITIES BEYOND WILDEST IMAGINATION. Tattooed, emaciated corpses were stacked like cordwood. Twenty-one thousand prisoners were liberated by the Americans, but had nowhere to go, and remained at the camp. For months before liberation, the volunteers read with interest, the prisoners' daily diet had been a piece of bread and a liter of thin soup. By May 2, the papers were speculating that Hitler was dead, but for the forty-three thousand victims of Buchenwald, it was too late.

For years, much of the world had willfully declined to believe the worst reports coming from death camp escapees and frantic Jewish activists. Even as the first crematories were discovered in 1945, the American newspapers repeated the Nazi story that they were only for disposing of prisoners who had died while performing slave labor—a horrifying enough explanation. By the time

Buchenwald was liberated, it was becoming impossible to deny the true nature of the Nazi camps. An article in the *Minneapolis Star Journal* entitled "Where Life Is Cheap," on April 23, 1945, described for the readers of the Twin Cities a lampshade made from human skin found at Buchenwald. A decorative wall hanging for the commandant's wife was made from the chest of an inmate. A former prisoner of the camp told the reporter, "It's just another instance of the lack of value the Nazis put on human life. They used humans as guinea pigs in experiments on typhus treatments. They'd destroy the hearing of a prisoner, or put out an eye, and leave him like that for weeks. Then they'd try to restore his sight or hearing. Sometimes they failed; sometimes they succeeded, but the experiment always ended with the victim's execution." The newspapers were still not describing the camps as a systematic effort to eliminate the Jewish people. Instead, in most reports, Jews just appeared as one group of many abused in the camps, if they were mentioned specifically at all.

Max Kampelman managed to fight through the hunger and slog through his law school courses with the dogged determination that had marked his entire, earnest young life. As starvation advanced, most gave up their academic ambitions. Not Max. The new "buddy" requirements in the wake of Watkins' cheating made it that much harder to attend class. Kampelman persevered. The psychologists noted with interest that despite showing typical physical deterioration, Max complained about the effects of hunger far less than his peers. They also noted that a girl Max had been romantically interested in during the control phase left his thoughts soon after the beginning of the starvation. The psychologists tracked three "drives" they considered fundamental to human beings—concern with food, desire for sex, and a need for activity. With all the volunteers, as with Max, interest in the opposite sex was among the first casualties of hunger.

The news of the Nazi atrocities caused twinges of conscience for Max, but he remained resolute in his pacifism. His left-leaning politics made him a firm believer that war was a tool of capitalism and business interests, fought and suffered by the poor. Beyond the political justification, Max believed unabashedly in "the power of love," the idealistic belief that only through man's love for his fellow man would civilization grow beyond its worst tendencies. It was a philosophy that Max could discuss without embarrassment with his CPS comrades, most of whom shared similar beliefs, whether sprung from the Sermon on the Mount or the writings of Gandhi. What the Nazis had done was unforgivable, but Max was still unwilling to say that war was the answer.

Never one to pass on a speaking engagement, even in the third week of starvation, Max articulated these beliefs at a March 3, 1945, speech to the Cosmopolitan Club on campus. The student group, whose goal was to promote international understanding, was conducting a program on conscientious objection and had asked Max to participate. Max addressed his hunger in passing: "You saw I ate my own sandwiches rather than your fine food, and I assure you that it is no reflection on your food; it's just that I'm one of the starvation guinea pigs." In a speech that echoed many of the arguments used by the CPS union organizers in Big Flats, New York, Max went on to describe what he saw as some fundamental problems with the CPS system.

"For the first time in American life, civilians are being conscripted to perform work for the government without receiving any salary for that work, without having compensation provided for them in case of injury during their work, without any provisions being made for their dependents. Such a state of affairs is a fork of involuntary servitude and violates the thirteenth amendment and further in substance punished American citizens for their religious convictions—a violation of the 1st amendment." The members of the Cosmopolitan Club hung on every word from the hungry-looking New York radical.

Henry Scholberg, too, persevered through the first half of the starvation phase to achieve a personal goal: playing Cléonte in the Molière play staged by the University's French club. Just as Max found peace of mind in his law classes, Henry was grateful for the distraction of learning his lines and rehearsal. He badly missed his parents, who were still in India. At the University of Illinois, he had been glad that their great distance insulated him from a conflict over his pacifist choice. The intervening years had replaced that with a simple longing to see his folks. The last time he saw them had been in 1939, when he waved good-bye to them from the deck of the *President Taft*.

Letters seldom came. Henry hoped that the war was to blame, and not his father's bitterness over his son's decision to become a CO. Because of their separation, they had never really had the chance to discuss the issue man to man. Henry hoped they were safe; he hoped they still loved him. His worst fears seemed to grow along with his hunger, at times keeping him awake at night in the dark barracks.

Although news was hard to come by, Henry knew that India was in chaos. Operating under the principle that the enemy of my enemy is my friend, Subhash Chandra Bose formed the Indian National Army to fight the British alongside the Nazis. Henry's hero, Gandhi, had tried to use support of the British war effort as leverage to gain Indian independence, but could secure no concessions. Churchill angrily said that he wasn't fighting the war "to preside over the liquidation of the British Empire." On August 9, 1942, Gandhi was arrested after the country was rocked by proindependence rallies. After seven months of incarceration, Gandhi decided in response to resort to a tactic that had worked for him in the past—the hunger strike.

He began the strike on February 10, 1943, at the Aga Khan Palace in Poona, where he was confined. For twenty-one days, he consumed only water supplemented with a small amount of lime juice and salt. Gandhi was seventy-four years old at the time. Several times during the strike attending physicians were certain he would die. Gandhi persevered somehow, and on the morning of March 3, he ended his fast, with prayers, hymns, a reading from the *Bhagavad Gita,* and a glass of orange juice.

Churchill, who had once called Gandhi "a miserable little old man," was unimpressed, convinced that someone must have been sneaking the Mahatma food during his "various fasting antics." Over the twenty-one-day duration of the fast, Gandhi dropped from 109 pounds to 91 pounds—a 16.5 percent weight loss—or a slightly smaller percentage than the men of the starvation experiment would lose in their first three months.

Gandhi was far from the only hungry man in India. While the British government had strictly regulated the food market at home with great success, they had allowed market forces to ravage the Indian food supply, in part to avoid offending the Indian upper classes who were their last supporters on the subcontinent. As supplies dwindled and inflation soared, food became priced out of reach for millions of Indians. The result was the 1943 Bengal Famine, which killed on the order of three million people, although the exact number will never be known. This indirect result of the war was the worst famine ever in a country with a long, sad history of epic hunger.

With Gandhi starving in jail, legions of Indians fighting for Hitler, and rampant starvation in Bengal, it was near anarchy in India, and no one knew what would happen next. The Molière play was a genteel, welcome refuge for Henry from his worst fears about the faraway country where his parents still lived.

Henry focused his efforts on his monologue, twelve lines near the middle of the play. He was aware that the starvation was affecting his concentration, and he worried that he would flub the speech. On stage, on opening night, in perfect French, Henry delivered the lines flawlessly. Everyone in the audience noted his believable sadness, his heartfelt weariness:

> *I display for a certain person all the ardor and affection conceivable. I love only her in all the world; I have her alone in my thought; she has all my devotion, all my desires, all my joy; I speak only of her, I think only of her, I dream only of her, I breathe only for her; and here is the fit reward for so much love! I pass two days without seeing her, which are to me two frightful centuries; I meet her only by chance; and at the sight my heart is utterly transported. My joy manifests itself upon my countenance. Ravished with delight, I fly to her; and the faithless one turns her face from me, and passes grimly by, as if she had never seen me in her life!*

Henry basked in the applause. He didn't confess to a soul that it was not a lost love he visualized while delivering the lines. Nor the parents he hadn't seen in over five years. Henry's lost loves were fresh bread, blueberry pie, the aromatic curries of his youth.

When Gandhi began his twenty-one-day hunger strike in 1943, he had obvious political reasons. In India, where the populace was never far removed from their last devastating famine, Gandhi's self-starvation carried great symbolic weight. The British, concerned greatly about the consequences of a martyred Gandhi, called the act political blackmail. When asked himself, however, Gandhi always justified his fasts in religious, Hindu terms. "My religion teaches me that, whenever there is distress which one cannot remove, one must fast and pray," he wrote. "A genuine fast cleanses the body, mind and soul. It crucifies the flesh and to that extent sets the soul free." Also: "I believe there is no prayer without fasting and no real fast without prayer."

Consuming food is perhaps our most tangible link to the physical world. It should be no surprise, then, that most of the world's religions have at times seen the self-denial of food as a highly spiritual act, a step towards breaking the bonds of the physical world and growing closer to God. Celibacy is similarly practiced by the religious devout of many cultures, another rejection of a primal physical need. The drive for activity is rejected by those who spend their days in quiet, prayerful meditation. It is interesting that monastic orders of all religions seem to police the same three "drives" of concern to Dr. Keys—food, sex, and activity. The CPS, without paying its members, even enforced a vow of poverty, of sorts.

The volunteers of the starvation experiment would have been familiar with Christianity's extensive ties to fasting. Fasting in the Old Testament occurred frequently, and for a variety of reasons. David fasted for seven days as an appeal to the Lord while his child by Bathsheba lay dying (2 Samuel 12:16). Ahab, King of Samaria, fasted as a penance for the killing of Naboth (1 Kings 21:27). The Israelites fasted for seven days in mourning when Saul and his three sons were killed by the Philistines (1 Chronicles 10:12). The writers—and readers—of the Old Testament were well aware of the holy nature of a fast, in its denial of earthly pleasures. Significantly, Adam and Eve were cast from paradise for breaking a kind of fast.

Jesus fasted in the wilderness for forty days and forty nights before being tempted by the devil. Jesus responded, "Man shall not live by bread alone," a favorite passage of the test subjects.

In the very early Christian church, desert monks gained fame and respect for their rigorous fasting, fasting that would last in some cases for years. In the fourth century, John the Hermit in the Egyptian desert prayed for three years and ate only the Eucharist on Sundays. Another renowned desert monk from the same era, Antony, ate only a meal of bread, salt, and water once per day. To their followers, the ability to survive on little or no food seemed to be strong evidence of the hand of God. One of the reasons that the monks advocated fasting was that it reduced sexual desires, another tie to the wicked, physical world. It was a side effect of hunger that the Minnesota subjects would have affirmed.

Later in church history, the ability to go without food was an important sign of holiness for a number of Christian saints. In the fifteenth century, Joan of Arc amazed her comrades in arms by eating only a few pieces of bread dipped in wine, even after the most rigorous battles. Saint Teresa of Avila in the sixteenth century fasted regularly and advocated this practice to enhance the practice of prayer. In an extreme example of "conquering the body," Saint Catherine of Siena stopped eating, drinking, and sleeping. She died of dehydration in 1380.

The official church would eventually come to eye these ascetics with more suspicion than reverence. They claimed a direct tie to the divine that made the priestly classes nervous. Nonetheless, many Christian churches would retain at least a symbolic fast in their liturgy over the centuries. Catholics, for example, were to abstain from meat on Fridays until the 1960s, and are still expected to practice meat abstention during Lent.

Keys had speculated that Asian religions might contribute to the higher resistance to cannibalism in the East, despite endemic famine. Part of the assertion might have been due to Keys' fondness for Asian culture. He had learned Chinese as a young man and traveled to Asia as a college student. There was also his practiced, intellectual distaste for Christianity. In any case, Keys diplomatically avoided pointing out the corollary to his Asian theory, that Christians were more likely to succumb to cannibalism because Christianity had attached a high symbolic value to the eating of flesh. Christ said, "Whoso eateth my flesh, and drinketh my blood, hath eternal life" (John 6:54). In some liturgies, particularly Roman Catholic, it was required for worshippers to believe that on the altar the communion wafer was not a symbol but had turned into the literal flesh of Christ. Interestingly, taking communion in these churches was normally preceded by fasting.

The Protestant churches from which most of the volunteers came had by and large rejected fasting, at least as a formal part of religious life. Nonetheless, these men who had grown up in deeply religious homes were certainly aware of the many mentions of fasting in the Bible that most read from every day. The Sermon on the Mount, cited by so many of the men as a primary spiritual inspiration, gives instructions on how to fast (Matthew 6:16). In addition, the guinea pigs might have independently reached the conclusion reached by so many monks and holy men throughout the ages, that by denying the body food they would be rejecting worldly things and reaching for the divine. It was a hopeful thought for religious young men as the experiment reached its halfway point.

Like Henry, Sam Legg also had a personal interest in news from the war zone. His mother's side of the family still lived in France. He did receive a tattered letter from his grandmother that had somehow crossed the battle lines and the Atlantic and made it into his hands inside Memorial Stadium. His grandmother, in elegant French, made no attempt to camouflage the fear and the deprivation that faced them in Grenoble. Nestled in the French Alps, only fifty miles from Geneva, Grenoble had been spared the worst battle scars. Still, the Gestapo was a visible presence and had turned neighbor against neighbor by recruiting collaborators. Food was in critically short supply. Sam thought of what remained of his pitiful family—his brother the worst, a drunken scoundrel. His ancestors under the boot heels of the Nazis. His mother, weak and dependent on an absent son. Even his sister, he worried, was wasting her life staying at home to take care of their mother. And here he was, indulging himself in a little altruistic starvation for the sake of science and his fellow man. Like Henry, Sam found it terrible to contemplate an imperiled family that he couldn't help, and couldn't even talk to.

The war in Europe ended at 5:01 PM Central time, on May 8, 1945, at the beginning of the thirteenth week of starvation. President Truman tempered the jubilation somewhat by reminding Americans that the war was only "half won"—the war against Japan loomed large in everyone's mind. Truman also said in the first line of his address to the nation, "I only wish Franklin D. Roosevelt had lived to witness this day." The news was punctuated by another front-page story that said that Hitler's dead body had been reportedly found in Berlin. In downtown Minneapolis, the massive central air-raid siren atop Northwestern National Bank wailed in celebration.

The mood in the lab was more subdued. The outside interests of the guinea pigs were starting to dwindle and die. On VE day, Marshall Sutton failed to mention the end of the war in Europe at all in his diary. His entry for May 8 begins with a small "132 3/4," his weight, down from an original 165.8 pounds. He goes on to say that "It would make a great psychological difference to our meal conversation & spirit if we did not wait in line so long before eating." The men who had volunteered to starve themselves to aid the victims of war found their interest in the war almost completely erased by hunger. Their world had shrunk to include only the stadium and the meal line at Shevlin Hall.

The other volunteers began to notice Sam Legg's strange behavior before the scientists did. In the barracks, he began collecting cookbooks, reading the recipes, and staring at the pictures of food with almost pornographic fascination. He was agitated in the meal lines, as they all were. More frequently than the rest of them, Legg's angst erupted into hostility. He jealously protected his place in line, and complained often and loudly that the women working the meal line weren't taking their jobs seriously enough. Once, while dishing steamed potatoes onto Legg's tray, one of the servers dropped her serving spoon. She had to walk back to the kitchen to retrieve another. During the delay, which didn't last more than thirty seconds, Legg began smashing his tray against the counter, saying "goddamn it, goddamn it, goddamn it." Legg had been regarded as one of the unofficial leaders of the group, and his evident deterioration was disturbing to them all.

His behavior soon came to the attention of the scientists. For weeks, it had been known that Legg liked to be left alone at meals, hovering over his tray at the end of the table, focused purely on eating. Because of his self-imposed isolation at meal times and because the other volunteers were engrossed in their own meals, it took a few minutes on that day for the others to notice that at the end of the table, Legg's behavior had taken another strange turn.

He had combined all the food on his tray into one pile. He then took his fork and stirred and smashed it all together, the thimble-fuls of fish chowder, spaghetti, peas, and potatoes, until it was a homogenous dark gray-greenish paste on his plate. He then salted and peppered the amalgamation until it was crusted with season-ing—the men were allowed salt and pepper in unlimited quanti-ties. Legg then began joylessly eating his creation.

The other volunteers, preoccupied with food as they were, stared open mouthed at Legg as he ate the disgusting concoction. When he had scraped every morsel off his plate, he then picked it up and licked it noisily until not a molecule of food remained. The slurping noise was so loud that it made the other men wince, but Legg continued, unaware or unconcerned with the discomfort he was causing his fellow guinea pigs.

Ancel Keys noted with some concern the psychological deterioration of the men. They had already lost one: Watkins. Two others, Willoughby and Plaugher, were each chewing forty packs of gum a day. Sam Legg's strange dining habits were disturbing the other men. The news of victory in Europe hardly cheered the men at all. The buddy system inconvenienced everybody, making it harder to enjoy what few pleasures there were left to them; it also seemed to signal a depressing collective collapse of will power. The old pep talk about all the good they were doing for the refugees of Europe seemed to motivate the men less and less. They didn't want to know how many people were starving in Holland—they wanted to know how many minutes until the next meal, how many days until rehabilitation.

Keys and his psychologists dutifully tried to quantify the misery of the men. On the lengthy inventory of fifty complaints that the men regularly completed, the number of complaints had risen sharply, from 6.6 on average during the control period to 15.1 at S12. The sex drive was determined to have dropped slightly more than the drive for activity, while the hunger drive had predictably soared. The men were asked regularly to rate a series of symptoms on a scale from -5 to +5, indicating the magnitude of increase or decrease from "normal." At S12, the men ranked "Appetite" with the biggest increase, followed closely by "Tiredness." While the food served was considerably more bland than the food of the control period, the hungry men also judged that the "Palatability of Food" had shot upwards since the beginning of the experiment. Ambition, self-discipline, mental alertness, concentration, and comprehension had all dropped in the self-evaluation.

While the discomfort of the men was entirely predictable, Keys still wondered about the overall collapse of morale. While Watkins had been exceptionally weak, Keys worried that he might have been just the canary in the coal mine, the first to succumb to an eventually widespread neurosis. Keys decided that a morale booster was in order. He decided to have a "relief meal" on May 26, near the end of the fifteenth week of starvation, and the twenty-seventh week overall. He allowed the men to pick the foods for the meal. The guinea pigs voted for the items they had been fantasizing about for three months. Keys carefully measured the calories for each food item, the percentage of protein and the precise vitamin content. In some cases he reduced quantities to keep the total number of calories in a reasonable range. Nonetheless, the relief meal served that day was largely just as the men had chosen. The meal they selected:

Grapefruit juice, 100 grams
Bacon, 10 grams
1 egg
Bread with butter and honey, 135 grams
Milk, 600 grams
Fruit punch, 100 grams
Chicken, 70 grams
Dressing, 70 grams
Potatoes, 150 grams
Gravy, 60 grams
Corn, 90 grams
Carrot salad, 80 grams
Strawberries, 90 grams
Baking powder biscuits, 70 grams
Celery, 10 grams
Peanut butter, 13 grams
Minced ham, 23 grams
Jelly roll, 30 grams
1 Orange

There it was, 2,366 glorious calories in one meal, compared to the 1,570 calories per day they had been consuming. The men absolutely loved the meal, each morsel made more enjoyable by their hunger and by the three months that had passed without tasting their favorite foods. Halfway through the meal, the solemnity that had begun to mark their meal times fell away, and they were joking, laughing, and once again beginning to remember the altruistic motives that had brought them to Memorial Stadium in the first place. George Ebeling stood and raised his glass of 100 grams of fruit punch and pompously quoted Shakespeare: "Small cheer and great welcome makes a merry feast." Such was the cheer of the men that his theatrics barely annoyed them.

Not a scrap of food remained on the trays as they finished the wonderful meal, just crumpled napkins, empty bowls, forks and spoons—and orange peel. The jocular conversation around the table slowed as all the men at once seemed to realize that while the natural time had come to return their trays and leave Shevlin Hall, this one potentially edible item remained uneaten. None of them could bring themselves to throw it away. The idea came to them collectively. They picked up the orange peel and ate it, every one of them. It was leathery but meaty in a pleasant way—the men craved bulk. The taste was slightly orangey and less astringent than they had expected.

Keys was furious when he found out. The orange peel was not part of the calculations he had carefully made. Who even knew what the nutritional content of the stuff was? Orange peel was in none of the standard nutritional tables. He ranted about the incident to his staff while they tried to keep their smiles hidden.

The next day, a Sunday, the men returned to their two meal, 1,570 calorie per day regimen. Keys was satisfied as he looked back on the first half of the experiment. They had lost one man, sure, and that still irked him. No one was seriously ill, though, and the thirty-five remaining men seemed just as resolute as when he had interviewed them months before. The continuing physical deterioration of the men, while distressing, was in many ways as mathematical and deliberate as a parabolic curve. Dr. Keys knew that over the second half of the experiment, the psychological journey of the men would be far less predictable.

CHAPTER SIX

———◄०►———

THE STIGMATA OF STARVATION

EARL WEYGANDT was the next to go.

Weygandt was from Clarksville, Michigan, a small farm town halfway between Lansing and Grand Rapids, one of eight children in a prosperous Disciples of Christ home. Before the starvation experiment, he had worked at CPS Camp 116, a Brethren Service Committee camp that ran tests on milk and dairy cows in College Park, Maryland. His work there so inspired him that he decided to make nutrition his calling after the war. The starvation experiment was a chance to pursue that vocation early.

He appeared to adjust wonderfully to life in Minneapolis. He was smart, funny, and charismatic. Before the buddy system, he landed a well-paying job as a bookkeeper in a Minneapolis cooperative grocery store. He told the other guinea pigs that he never felt tempted to cheat, "even when I handle food." He did indeed seem to be one of the strongest members of the group. His strong will and his copious pocket change were envied in equal measure by the other volunteers.

Keys was less confident about the strength of Weygandt's character. To Keys, Weygandt's oft-expressed self-confidence was a mark of insecurity. The man's diary was simplistic and Pollyannaish. His frequent use of exclamation points in particular annoyed Keys. His stated purpose in life: "To do that which is right in the sight of God our maker, trying always to advance His kingdom on earth. Truly, life is worthwhile!" In his opinion of Weygandt, Keys exercised his tendency to equate religious devotion with simple-mindedness.

Keys also had his trusted MMPI graphs with which to evaluate the inner Weygandt. Weygandt rated highly on the test's "Lie" scale, a strand of the test designed to ferret out those who were being untruthful in their responses. Weygandt also seemed to regard himself in his test answers as nearly perfect. On the MMPI, Weygandt indicated that he always told the truth, liked everyone he knew, and never felt like swearing. Keys noted dryly, "such an individual must be singularly resistant to self-revelation."

It was a diagnosis Keys took no pleasure in. He had originally wanted forty men in the study, but could only find thirty-six volunteers that met the minimum requirements. Given Watkins' collapse, each man lost now would represent an almost three percent loss in the study's total data. Any such loss would also reduce the statistical reliability of every test they ran because of the smaller sample size. Keys did not want to lose another man.

In week seven of the starvation phase, before the implementation of the buddy system, Weygandt was alone in the grocery store downtown, finishing up his ledger entries for the night. The store was blissfully quiet. Being alone was a rare treat for a guinea pig, with their group meals and communal barracks. Solitude was something that Weygandt had learned to treasure about his job. Those few quiet minutes at the end of a busy day were more valuable than his much-envied pay. Heavy snow and bitter cold had kept customers away all day. Weygandt finished his paperwork early and waited for the clock to strike nine. He sat peacefully on his stool behind the counter. At the far end of the store, beyond the shelves of Spam, evaporated milk, and Sunnyfield Rice Puffs, a Regulator clock ticked through the final minutes of the workday. Weygandt sighed. A wind gust rattled the front door in its frame, ringing the dangling bell as if to announce the arrival of a phantom customer.

Weygandt suddenly realized that his hand held a cookie.

He looked down. His hand was moving of its own independent will. He was helpless to stop it. He shoved the cookie in his mouth. It tasted wonderful.

He shoved two more cookies in his mouth. A sack of popcorn was also within reach and he ate that next. Finally, he ate two overripe bananas that he had been planning to throw in the trash on his way out the door.

With a final swallow of gooey brown banana, Weygandt regained control of himself, and again looked at the Regulator clock. Just three minutes had passed.

Earl Weygandt locked up the store in a panic, and ran back to the lab, sliding and falling three times on the icy sidewalks as he hurtled through Minneapolis. In the lab, he found Dr. Brozek, the experiment's chief psychologist. Brozek was finishing up his notes for the day at his desk, his face lit from beneath by the single bulb of his desk lamp. Brozek looked up as Weygandt burst into the room, alarmed to see one of the test subjects so upset. Weygandt was gasping for breath. His messy hair was soaked with sweat and melting snow. Some of the other guinea pigs peered in the office after Weygandt, concerned and curious to see him running in there like that. He acted in his haste and his fear as if he were being chased by an angry mob.

"What is wrong, young man?" asked Brozek, in a thick Czech accent. Josef "Yashka" Brozek had only been in the United States since 1939. He had been a "psychotechnologist" at the Bata Shoe Factory in Zlin before fleeing the war. He had been at the University of Minnesota ever since, and, along with Henry Longstreet Taylor, had become one of Keys' most trusted lieutenants.

"I . . . I had a mental blackout," said the agitated Weygandt. He was on the verge of crying. "I ate some cookies, some popcorn, and . . ."

Brozek raised an eyebrow. A lifetime spent in clinical environments had honed his instincts, and he deftly shoved himself away from his desk just as Weygandt vomited the forbidden fruit upon it. Several guinea pigs rushed in to assist the agitated Weygandt and to help Brozek clean up. When the situation had somewhat stabilized, Brozek dutifully reported Weygandt's violations to Dr. Keys, who was attempting to enjoy a rare quiet evening with his family along the shores of Lake Owasso.

Just as he had with Watkins, Keys hoped that the incident would be isolated, and that Weygandt could be kept in the experiment. Weygandt assured the doctor, and everyone else who would listen, that he had learned his lesson, and that he was once again the most self-controlled member of the experiment. He even argued that he was in a stronger position, having gotten the cheating out of his system. Like Watkins before him, though, Weygandt's weight soon began to veer from his predictive curve. The scientists, unable to catch him cheating, slashed his diet in order to bring his weight down. Weygandt's status as a leader of the group disappeared. With the implementation of the buddy system, he had to give up his plum job at the co-op grocery. Weygandt's self-assured façade began falling away in chunks. In the end, though, it wouldn't be cheating that brought about Weygandt's removal from the experiment.

Like all of the volunteers, Weygandt had become morbidly fascinated with his own bodily functions. One volunteer, Carlyle Frederick, went to the doctors alarmed that he hadn't had a bowel movement in ten days. Keys told him not to worry, his starving body was just metabolizing every crumb of food he consumed, leaving no waste behind. The men had the opposite problem with urination. They all took frequent advantage of the rule that allowed them black coffee and water in unlimited quantities, an opportunity to put something in their mouths and stomachs. In addition, many of the men had begun to indulge in "souping" their meals, mixing everything in drinking water to create the illusion of an increased quantity. The result was "polyuria," urine production in spectacular quantities. During the control period, the men had on average produced 1.33 quarts of urine per day. By S12, that had risen to 1.86 quarts. Their production peaked at an amazing 2.58 quarts of transparent, colorless urine per day, as their coffee and water consumption soared.

Weygandt realized that he was paying more attention to his body than normal. He also realized that he had already made a name for himself as a cheater, and was reluctant to attract further attention. So he waited weeks before telling any of the scientists that his urine appeared to be changing colors.

At first he wasn't even sure. He saw just a slight darkish tint as his urine splashed against the white porcelain on the back of the urinal. Weygandt watched it closely as the days passed and his urine darkened to the same color as iced tea. At that point, he was forced to mention the problem to the staff. He was urinating blood.

He felt almost as if he were confessing cheating again, as if he had somehow willed the blood into his urine in order to escape the laboratory.

Dr. Keys refused to link the problem definitively to either the starvation or Weygandt's neurosis. Indeed, Weygandt had had a similar urological problem years before. Keys wrote that the problem was "of obscure etiology." It was a serious medical problem nonetheless, and Keys was forced to drop another man from the experiment. It was the eighteenth week of starvation.

Weygandt seemed to share Keys' feeling that the blood in his urine somehow represented a personal failure. He wrote in his diary, *Sense of failure was almost predominant! Mentally, emotionally, and physically, I was a mess. My first thought was escape from it all! Try and forget it as just a bad dream!* No doubt the frequent exclamation points annoyed Keys almost as much as losing another three percent of his data set.

Weygandt stayed at Unit 115 to help in the kitchen until the end of the experiment. Like Watkins, within a few days of normal meals, all symptoms, mental and physical, disappeared.

They were down to thirty-four.

———

While Victory in Europe had arrived on May 8, the constant news from Japan proved that the war was far from over. Every day's newspaper brought with it reports of some massive assault or air raid the Japanese had endured, but surrender seemed nowhere in sight. On the editorial page of the *Minneapolis Star Journal,* a political cartoon of a buck-toothed, near-sighted caricature labeled "Nip" was shown hanging himself with his pledge to "fight to the finish." While the war in the East dragged on, at least the lists of liberated prisoners in the newspaper were now longer than the lists of local casualties. It was a small sign of hope that went unnoticed inside the South Tower.

"What happened to Earl?" asked Bob Willoughby. He and Jim Plaugher were walking through downtown Minneapolis on a bitterly cold day. It was late May, but so far they had seen only the briefest glimpses of spring weather. At least they no longer had to dodge the giant mountains of snow being pushed along the streets by the monstrous snowplows. They were trying to get five miles of walking in before the sun set, which would put them on track for their twenty-two miles for the week.

"Don't know," said Plaugher. Willoughby wished the scientists could hear these conversations. He knew they thought his friend Plaugher evasive in interviews, but it was really just Plaugher's nature. Willoughby was Plaugher's best friend in the experiment, the man he most trusted in Minnesota, and even for him talking to Plaugher was usually like talking to a cigar store Indian. Willoughby had come to admire his friend's stubborn refusal to gab. Unlike almost everyone else in the experiment, Plaugher was not in love with the sound of his own voice.

"I heard Earl was cheating again," said Willoughby. "But somebody else heard that he had some kind of infection."

Plaugher shrugged noncommittally and shoved his gloved hands further into his pockets.

"They still think we're cheating, don't they?" asked Willoughby after a few more steps. Plaugher stopped abruptly, his countenance darkening.

"Why do you say that?"

"Because!" said Willoughby. "You know why. Because we're not losing weight like the others. Because we're eating less than anyone, but we're not losing weight on the curve."

"Well, there's got to be some explanation other than cheating, right?" asked Plaugher. "I mean . . . you're not cheating are you?"

"Of course not!" Willoughby was shocked that his friend would even think at this point that it was possible.

"Good," said Plaugher. "Because I think that would be about the worst thing a guy could do here." He resumed walking.

Willoughby knew he wouldn't be getting an apology so he tried to let it go. Plaugher was just feeling the effects of hunger, that's all, and he hadn't meant anything by the accusation.

In fact, a half mile later, Plaugher did consider apologizing. At that moment, though, the pair walked by an overflowing garbage can that even in the cool air reeked of decay. Plaugher felt an almost overwhelming urge to root through the can and eat the rancid waste as fast as he could. Fighting that temptation took all his strength, and the apology to his friend was lost in the struggle.

Max Kampelman filed into the small auditorium along with the rest of the volunteers. Every one of them carried a blanket that they folded up and placed on their chairs—a loss of natural padding was one of the many uncomfortable side effects of wasting away. Sitting for any length of time had become painful, as body fat dropped from an average of almost 14 percent to about 5 percent. The guinea pigs had gotten in the habit of bringing along some sort of cushion wherever they went.

The men filing into the auditorium were overdressed as well, wearing layers of shirts and sweaters despite the adequate heating of the room. They were cold all the time. Part of the body's desperate attempt to conserve energy was to lower the thermostat. As a result, body temperatures for the volunteers had dropped from the normal 98.6°F to an average of 95.8°F. In one of the most striking changes in the experiment, the average heart rate had slowed from an average of 55 beats per minute in control to just 35 beats per minute, barely one beat every two seconds. Their bodies were trying frantically to conserve every calorie. The lowest recorded pulse rate was a startling 28 beats per minute. It belonged to Henry Scholberg.

Max realized as he walked in that he had not seen the room so full in weeks. The education program had been used to recruit many of the volunteers just a year before, but in their hunger, lectures were now seen as something to be endured rather than an opportunity to learn. In addition to the physical discomfort associated with sitting, the volunteers didn't have the energy or the interest to listen to long dissertations from relief workers or professors. The laboratory staff had gotten into the habit of warning visiting speakers that their audience would be perhaps less attentive than they were accustomed to. The speakers were encouraged to bring up the subject of food whenever possible, the only topic that truly engaged the guinea pigs. The week before, a young assistant from the university's agricultural school came to discuss the innovative new uses for soybeans, and was surprised by the intensity of the questions he received from his gaunt audience.

Today's speaker was packing the room, despite the fact that he had nothing to say about food, nutrition, or the latest advances in soybeans. He was Norman Matoon Thomas, five-time Socialist candidate for president and ardent critic of the war.

Max Kampelman had actually shared a podium with the famous Socialist's brother, Evan Thomas, in pacifist rallies in New York City before the war. It was Evan's imprisonment in

World War I that led in part to Norman's adoption of pacifism. While none of the other guinea pigs had so direct a connection to Thomas, they all were anxious to hear a talk from the country's most famous (or notorious) pacifist.

Thomas had run for president in every election since 1928. In 1932, his best year, he had received 896,000 votes. That year he had spoken to huge, enthusiastic crowds that chanted his name across the country. Since then, the war and J. Edgar Hoover's efficient crusade against the left had taken their toll on the Socialist movement, and Thomas had learned to accept his place on the fringes of American politics. His votes dwindled with each election, as did the crowds for his speeches. With the start of World War II and his opposition to it, those crowds were now frequently hostile. He had become adept at dodging rotten eggs while finishing a prepared speech on the immorality of war.

While he was the flag bearer for the Socialist party in the United States, Norman Thomas was also the son and grandson of Presbyterian ministers on both sides. He had been a Presbyterian pastor himself before World War I. Indeed, with his dignified dark suit and neat, silver hair, he looked far more like a New England preacher than the wild-eyed Bolshevik he was often accused of being. He was a powerful speaker, and he knew well the language of the religious pacifist.

Unfortunately, despite his great oratorical skills and despite the great admiration most of the men in the laboratory had for him, Thomas's speech came too late in the experiment. He talked about the history of conscientious objection. He talked about his brother's prison sentence during the First World War. He talked about the problems with the current CPS system. All he got in return were blank stares from those guinea pigs who had managed to stay awake. Thomas was an experienced enough speaker to know that he had hopelessly lost his audience. He was much more fascinated by the skeletal young conscientious objectors than they were by him.

Thomas made a decision on the podium to cut his comments short. "Thank you for having me, and thank you for your service," he said. The men began to tiredly applaud. "I would still like to learn more about what you're doing here," he said. "I was wondering if I might stay here with you boys tonight?"

The staff ran the request by Keys. He admired the fact that a man in Thomas's position would volunteer to sleep on a cot in a room full of thirty-four starving, snoring young men; none of the other visiting speakers had asked to. Keys was also always looking for opportunities to boost morale. He approved the request, and a cot and clean sheets were hurriedly set up for their famous guest.

America's most infamous left-wing agitator spent a pleasant night in the barracks beneath the football stadium at the University of Minnesota. The men gathered around him, asking politely about his views on the war, politics, and pacifism. Somehow, the conversation would always come back to food.

Scholberg barely noticed the Thomas talk. He had come to Minnesota to escape the hospital and the craziness he felt growing inside him. Now the hunger was starting to crawl inside his head the same way the insane laughter of the inmates had in Maryland. In the food line, he insisted that everything he ate be served as hot as possible. He felt that his exhausted body could convert the heat from his food directly into energy. Henry was also drinking as many as fifteen cups of coffee per day. It did nothing to help Henry's growing problem with controlling his temper.

One day after the Thomas visit, Henry somehow ended up at the same table in Shevlin Hall as George Ebeling, a situation he normally avoided. Ebeling had become something of a scapegoat for the guinea pigs, with his overly dramatic ways and his insistence on being at the center of attention at all times. Many of the men when discussing their condition would punctuate their self-evaluation by saying, "well, at least I'm not as bad as Ebeling."

Henry was one of the last men in the food line that day, though, and there was nowhere else to sit. Henry weighed 121 pounds, down from his original weight of 145 pounds. He was cold all the time, his butt hurt when he sat for more than five minutes, and he found sleep didn't even offer him relief; he slept uncomfortably without the energy to turn over. The dinner that evening was Henry's least favorite: 250 grams of potato soup and 285 grams of turnip stew. All food tasted delicious to Henry at that point, but that particular supper seemed to him to be the least substantial of the three dinners they were served in rotation. Henry prayed before every meal, and that evening he asked God to keep George Ebeling's thespian mouth shut.

It was not to be. "So sharp are hunger's teeth," said George. He was looking straight ahead. As usual no one had chosen to sit across from him because of his frequent recitations. He was speaking in that peculiar fake British accent that he reserved for his most dramatic orations. "That man and wife draw lots who first shall die to lengthen life." Ebeling's loud voice annoyed Henry so much that his eye began to twitch.

There was an uncomfortable silence in Shevlin Hall as the guinea pigs realized collectively that the most annoying man in the experiment had somehow ended up sitting next to the most high-strung. They tried as a group to will silence upon Ebeling.

Henry shook off George's last comment. He tried to put himself into a state of yogic calm. He raised a watery spoonful of turnip stew to his mouth as George remembered another line.

"Let's leave this town; for they are hare-brain'd slaves . . . And hunger will enforce them to be more eager." George was speaking louder now, oblivious as always to the grating effect his dramatics had on everyone around him. Henry was grinding his teeth and staring straight ahead. He tried to remember the Sermon on the Mount, something Gandhi wrote, anything to keep him from killing a fellow human being, no matter how justified.

George was almost shouting now: "Woe, alas! What in, our house?"

"George?" said Henry. George looked over, surprised that he had been interrupted.

"Yes, Henry?"

Henry had very limited experience with profanity, moving as he had from a missionary school in India to his sister's house, to the Civilian Public Service, an organization run for and by the religiously devout. Fortunately, he had studied briefly at the knee of a cursing prodigy, the stowaway on the *President Taft*. "George, why don't you do us all a favor, and shut . . . your fucking . . . mouth."

Henry held his gaze until Ebeling finally looked away. Henry felt a momentary sense of triumph as he watched Ebeling look down at his tray. That exultation evaporated as he saw Ebeling's clear shame, and Henry realized that not only had he humiliated the man: he had ruined George's meal. That was the ultimate blasphemy in Shevlin Hall. While the others lingered over their sorry stew in typical fashion, trying to pretend nothing had happened, Ebeling hurriedly finished and left as soon as he could draft a "buddy" to return with him to the stadium. In his abject guilt, Henry found his meal ruined as well. He wondered if his outburst was yet another indication that he was losing his mind.

Henry vowed to apologize. Back in the barracks, he couldn't bring himself to face the man he had publicly humiliated. He wrote it down instead: *How many people have I hurt with my indifference, my grouchiness, my overbearing perversion for food? Please forgive me. I was crazy and I didn't know it.*

Like everything else, the incident in Shevlin made its way back to Keys and Brozek. They questioned Scholberg about it. Henry was, as always, forthright about his fears for his sanity. There was no need to parse answers, interpret dreams, or study MMPI graphs with Henry. "I am going crazy," he told them. He added for good measure that he often felt a compelling desire to smash and break things.

So far, though, Henry's only antisocial act had been a verbal outburst directed at George Ebeling, hardly a sign of encroaching lunacy. Keys was loath to lose another man's data. He and Brozek decided to keep Scholberg in, while continuing to watch him closely.

Henry, along with many others, saw his weight loss begin to plateau around the twentieth week of starvation. Unlike Willoughby and Plaugher, their stalled weight losses were entirely explicable and did not put them under suspicion of cheating. Henry and the other men were suffering from edema. The condition was, as Keys would put it, one of the chief "stigmata" of starvation.

Edema was a puffy swelling caused by retained water in the body. It occurred chiefly in the ankles and knees, but also in the face. Every morning, each subject found the side of his face that he had slept on swollen. Henry had a severe case. His legs were like elephant feet, virtually the same diameter all the way down from his knees to his toes. It became uncomfortable and then impossible for him to cram his feet into his normal shoes. When he pressed a fingertip against his shins, the indentation stayed, as if he had pressed his finger into clay. He would at times amuse himself by making a row of indentations run up his leg like buttons on a shirt.

While edema had been linked to famine for ages, the causes were obscure. Because it was such a conspicuous symptom of starvation, Keys would devote a full chapter to edema in his final study, where he mostly debunked the different theories that attempted to explain it. One school of thought held that famine edema was caused by increasing intercapillary pressure, pushing fluid from the blood into the interstitial space between cells. Others believed it was due to an increased permeability of the capillaries. Keys addressed all the theories in the book, dubious that any of them had it completely right. Edema was the body's ironic comment on starvation, a swelling caused by wasting away.

Edema also greatly complicated the weight loss calculations. As the body retained water, it made the weight loss slow, even as the affected subject continued to lose fat and tissue at the predicted rate. With no objective way to measure the percent of a man's weight caused by edema, Keys was forced to make educated guesses about individual diets and weight loss.

Sam Legg quit teaching his French course on the day in S21 when he was the only one who showed up at the squash court. Interest in the class had been waning for weeks. The men seemed less and less interested in preparing for real relief work. Sam's interest in teaching the class had been steadily dropping as well; he couldn't blame others for dropping out. It was hard to concentrate, but even more, it was hard to care. At one time, Sam had headed a group of the more activist volunteers who were agitating for a greater say in the operations of Unit 115. They felt a guinea pig council ought to be formed to have some control over the program—unthinkable by both the scientists and the Selective Service. The staff had not needed to suppress that incipient rebellion; with hunger it just withered away. The subjects had no interest in studying French, preparing for relief work overseas, or self-government. All they wanted was for their 255 grams of macaroni to be served hot and on time.

On June 22, 1945, during the twentieth week of starvation, the guinea pigs received another memorable visitor. He was a young army sergeant with first-hand knowledge of what hunger could do to a man.

The sergeant spent the morning with the staff, touring the lab, shaking hands, and watching the men run on the treadmill. He was in a new army uniform that was festooned with ribbons. Unlike a Hollywood war hero, however, his uniform hung on pointy shoulders, and his pants were cinched tightly around his narrow waist. His cheekbones were hollow. While he smiled through the tour, and laughed politely along with the staff, he had a somewhat haunted look in his eyes, as if the sight of so many young hungry men in close quarters brought back recent, disturbing memories. The sergeant's presence was less disruptive to the guinea pigs than previous visits by well-fed generals and admirals. The guinea pigs just saw another emaciated young man. Except for the uniform, he looked just like them.

They assembled in the auditorium to hear him speak before their evening meal. Some of the men were nervous when they heard they were to be addressed by a war hero. They were afraid he might challenge their pacifism, angrily explain to them the sacrifices he had made for their freedom. Even if he didn't say it, his presence was an uncomfortable reminder that others were dying for the freedom of religion that they had chosen to exercise. It was a paradox of which the men of the starvation experiment were well aware. When the soldier spoke, though, he didn't yell or excoriate. His voice was so quiet they had to strain to hear him at the front of the room.

"I was captured in December," he almost whispered. "During the Jerry breakthrough in Belgium. I weighed 190 pounds when they captured us." He laughed, as if he couldn't believe it himself, "I was fat, friends! Anyway, the first thing the Krauts did was take our boots and our socks—I don't know if this was to keep us from escaping, or because they needed the boots and socks. Probably both. Then they marched us for four days in just our galoshes. That was entirely without food. Finally, they gave us a loaf of bread for every four men. I wanted to save a little piece of mine for later, but I couldn't. I ate all of my share right then and there."

The guinea pigs nodded in recognition of the behavior. It was impossible not to like the former POW. They had grown so accustomed to talking only with scientists and with each other. The majority of speakers and visitors to the lab had been scientific or intellectual types. It was refreshing to hear from a plain-speaking, regular joe.

"Then, they loaded us into boxcars, and we took another four-day trip locked up like cattle. At the end of that, we hiked three miles up a mountain to Bad Orb Prison Camp. There we got our first hot meal—a bowl of grass soup."

"Most days after that, we got a ration of a tiny bit of oats, potatoes, a smudge of margarine, and some kind of tea. That was it." He paused. "I was there a hundred days and lost fifty pounds." He stopped for a minute and looked down at his feet. Telling the story seemed to have exhausted him. The guinea pigs were relieved when the GI looked up again, smiled and lifted his hands up. "So, I guess the reason I'm telling you all this is that I also used to hide food under my pillow and stare at pictures of bread like they were pinups of Betty Grable—I recognize your deviant behavior." The guinea pigs laughed. "So how about it— are you fellows ready to eat? You'll have to forgive my table manners, though. I've been a guest of the Nazis—the bastards." They walked together to Shevlin Hall.

They had been worried that a soldier would be an odd presence among them. But, because of his age and his experience with hunger, their similarities were far more pronounced than their differences. The soldier gustily ate his fish chowder, chuckling sympathetically as some of the men around him repeatedly diluted the soup with hot water.

Max Kampelman was sitting next to him. Max was eager to hear an eyewitness account of the situation in Europe. "Were there political prisoners at Bad Orb?" asked Max.

Just as the soldier began to answer, a solitary pea fell from Max's fork. Without hesitation, Max dove under the table and popped the pea in his mouth before it could be stepped on or lost.

When he came back up, he and the soldier resumed their conversation as if nothing unusual had happened.

All the men felt good to have him there. He was a reminder of the war, a reminder of what had brought them together in Minnesota. He was also a reminder that others had been through worse, and survived. It was a better meal because of his company.

On July 20, 1945, in the final week of starvation, Ancel Keys waited at Gate 27 for another military visitor, surprised at his own anxiety. He had welcomed higher-ranking military men to the lab before, beribboned generals and admirals curious about where this tiny fraction of the military budget was going. Keys was never intimidated by uniforms or titles, and had great confidence in his War Department connections, should some creaky general from Fort Snelling ever decide that Keys' work needed auditing. No, Keys was not nervous about welcoming an Army major to the Laboratory of Physiological Hygiene. He was nervous because this particular officer, Marvin Corlette, was a doctor, and had seen firsthand the starving victims of the Nazi concentration camps. He also happened to be the chief of the Civilian Nutrition Branch of the Army's Medical Corps. For the first time, Keys was about to bring a man through the lab with both the credentials and the experience to rigorously evaluate the starvation experiment.

Keys showed Major Corlette the barracks, Shevlin Hall, and their array of testing equipment. Corlette was more eager to get to the men. Keys watched from across the room as the major talked to them, took notes, and examined their swollen ankles. Keys wasn't about to ask this young major his opinion, but he listened closely to the major's questions and comments in an attempt to discern his frame of mind. Did he think that Keys had accurately recreated concentration camp–style famine? Or did he think the whole experiment was a circus, a dangerous, indulgent exercise in scientific showmanship? Major Corlette was civil and cheerful, but he left the laboratory without sharing his conclusions.

Keys was too busy to sit around and worry, but annoyance at the major's reticence stuck with him in the coming weeks. His curiosity about the major's opinion was finally satisfied when he got a letter from Corlette dated August 18 summarizing his visit to the lab.

Corlette began by describing the symptoms of the men: "Most had gaunt pinched faces and the peculiar sallow color that those of us who had seen the concentration camps had learned to associate at a glance with starvation." He then evaluated Keys' work as a whole: "Except for the absence of filth and secondary skin infections in the experimental subjects, it appears that the fundamental clinical pattern of partial starvation as we observed in Europe has been duplicated." Because Keys had been too proud to admit to anyone that Corlette's opinion mattered to him, he could take only private satisfaction in the evaluation.

Through all phases of the experiment, Max managed to complete those miscellaneous law school courses he needed, thanks to his own considerable will power and the assistance of countless anonymous "buddy" guinea pigs who agreed to sit through class with him. Several of his teachers, self-proclaimed radicals all, were disciples of Evron "Kirk" Kirkpatrick. Kirkpatrick was an Indiana farm boy turned Yale PhD, and was head of the University's social sciences department. Kirkpatrick had a knack for spotting and mentoring young talent, and he saw something that he liked in Max. He introduced Max to his circle of young protégés, including the thirty-four-year-old former pharmacist who had just been elected mayor of Minneapolis. His name was Hubert Humphrey.

Max's hard work had paid off. NYU accepted the University of

Minnesota credits, as expected, and Max applied for admission to the New York Bar. Admission was supposed to be automatic. For the first time, however, Max was to encounter a significant negative reaction to his pacifist stance. Weak from hunger, Max was about to face his biggest fight.

His chief antagonist was John G. Jackson, Vice Chairman of the New York Bar's Committee on Character and Fitness. He interpreted Max's conscientious objection as an unwillingness to "support and defend" the constitution of New York, part of the bar's oath. He referred Max to a similar case in Illinois where a CO had been refused admission to the bar. Ominously, the United States Supreme Court had upheld the state's right to reject the application in that case. As the delay lengthened, it appeared to Max that Jackson was intent on exercising a pocket veto over his application, delaying it into oblivion.

Never one to back away from a challenge, Max went on the attack, writing stacks of letters from the rickety desk and typewriter inside the barracks. In his letters to Jackson, Max argued politely but firmly the fine points of the Illinois case, stating that the court had merely upheld Illinois's right to deny admission to the bar. The court had not stated that COs could not, or should not, be admitted. Max wrote, "the decision, you will note, reaffirms *in dicta* the fact that a public official may take the oath of allegiance without promising to bear arms."

Already in possession of fine political instincts, Max wasn't willing to rely on legal arguments alone. He started calling and writing his friends. He had come to Minneapolis as a stranger; in fact, he had never before been west of Reading, Pennsylvania. Thanks to his natural charm, as well as his impressive work ethic, he had made influential friends who were interested in his success. Max got letters of recommendation from them all.

Max's advocates made up a diverse cast of characters, from the Jewish Peace Fellowship leader Rabbi Isador Hoffman to the atheist Ancel Keys, who wrote the committee that Max "proved

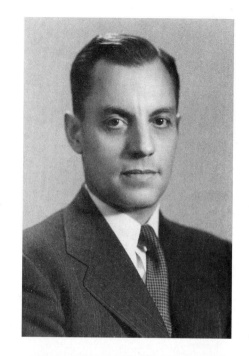

Dr. Ancel Keys in 1945, the year the starvation experiment ended. He was forty-one years old and already famous for inventing the army's K ration.
University of Minnesota Archives

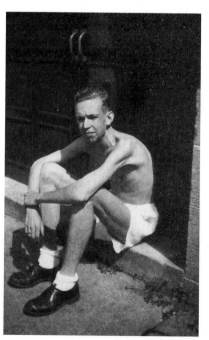

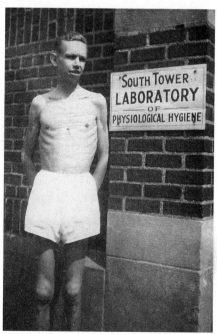

Henry Scholberg near the end of the experiment. His weight had dropped from 145 pounds to 117 pounds. Average caloric intake during the starvation phase was 1,570 calories per day, about half the amount required to maintain weight constant.
Courtesy of Henry Scholberg

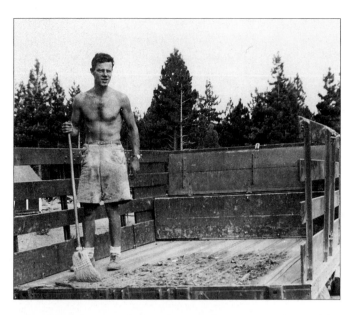

Sam Legg in 1942, before the experiment, at Civilian Public Service Camp #101 in Coleville, California. Many of the idealistic conscientious objectors found forestry work less than fulfilling, and sought out more challenging alternatives. *Courtesy of Sam Legg*

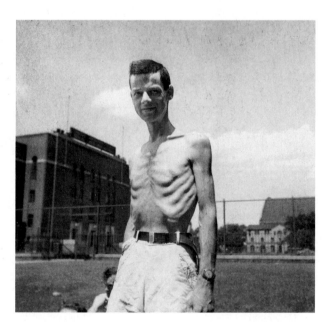

Wallace Kirkland photo of Sam Legg that appeared in the July 30, 1945 issue of *Life*. *Wallace Kirkland/Time & Life Pictures/Getty Images*

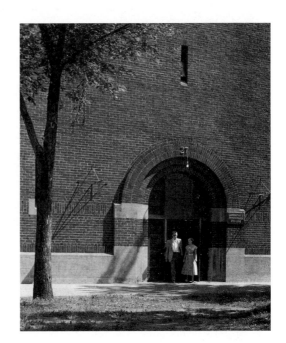

Gate 27, the entrance to the Laboratory of Physiological Hygiene. Originally intended as temporary quarters, the football stadium would become the lab's permanent home. *University of Minnesota Archives*

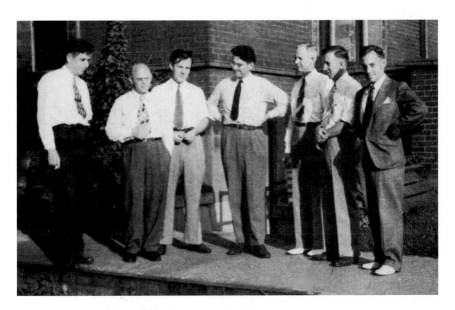

A rare photograph of the senior staff during the experiment. They are, from left to right: Drs. Henry Longstreet Taylor, Ernst Simonson, unknown, Josef Brozek, Austin Henschel, Olaf Mickelsen, and Ancel Keys.
Courtesy of Marshall Sutton

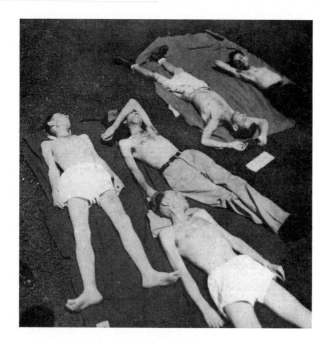

Test subjects sunning themselves near the end of the starvation phase, June 1945. Keeping warm was a constant struggle as body temperatures and pulse rates plummeted. *Wallace Kirkland/Time & Life Pictures/Getty Images*

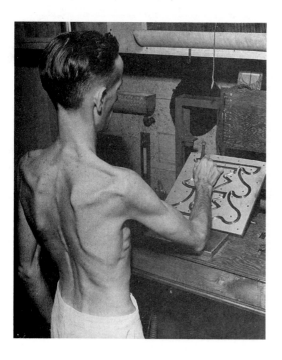

Charles Smith taking a test for dexterity, just of one of hundreds of tests Keys used to quantify the toll taken by starvation. As measured by this test, coordination deteriorated almost 22 percent during the starvation phase. Other attributes, such as hearing, actually improved. *Wallace Kirkland/Time & Life Pictures/Getty Images*

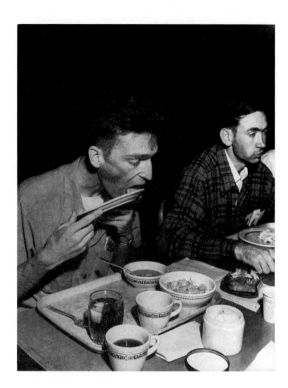

Bill Anderson licking his plate in the starvation phase, a common behavior. To his left is Dan Peacock. *Wallace Kirkland/Time & Life Pictures/Getty Images*

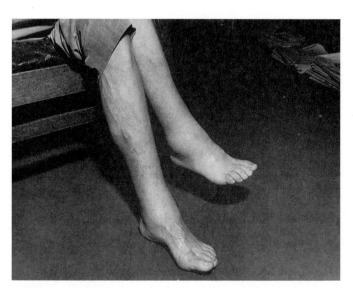

Henry Scholberg's legs, swollen by edema late in experiment. The condition, puzzling to the scientists and frustrating to the volunteers, may have been related to the massive quantities of water the test subjects consumed in an attempt to fill their stomachs. *Wallace Kirkland/Time & Life Pictures/Getty Images*

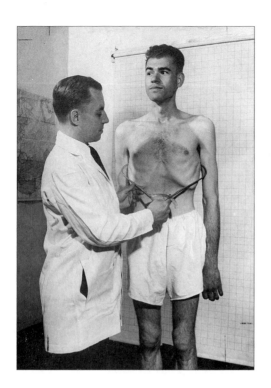

Ancel Keys measures the chest of James Plaugher for *Life* magazine. Plaugher was later thrown out of the experiment for cheating. *Wallace Kirkland/Time & Life Pictures/Getty Images*

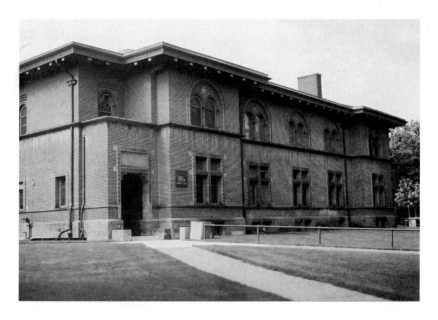

Shevlin Hall, where the Guinea Pigs took their meals. The two carefully measured meals per day during the starvation phase became events of almost sacramental importance. *Todd Tucker*

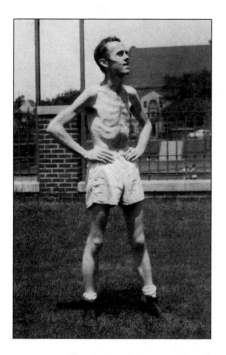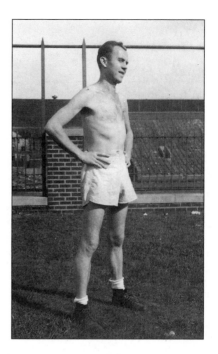

Dan Miller during the twenty-fourth week of starvation, and during the recovery period. Miller's 24.5 percent weight loss was typical. *Courtesy of Henry Scholberg*

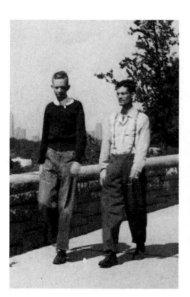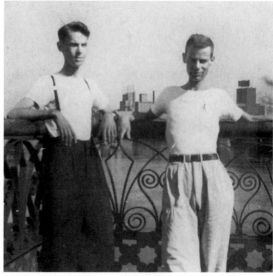

On left: Henry Scholberg and Ray Summers. *On right:* Donald Sanders and Sam Legg. All of the test subjects were required to walk twenty-two miles outdoors, every week. *Courtesy of Marshall Sutton*

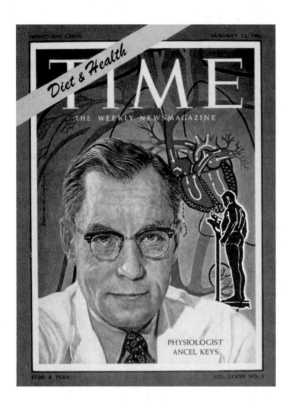

Ancel Keys on cover of *Time* magazine, January 13, 1961. He had become America's nutritionist laureate. The article discusses Keys' novel theory that cholesterol is linked to heart disease, but mentions nothing of the starvation experiment. *Time & Life Pictures/Getty Images)*

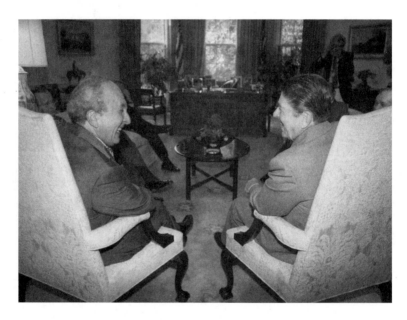

Max Kampelman laughing with President Ronald Reagan in the Oval Office in 1985. *Corbis/Tim Clary*

to be a highly reliable and conscientious man who comported himself well under the most rigorous and demanding circumstances." Another letter described Max's service in Minnesota to the Committee on Character: "By volunteering for this program Mr. Kampelman demonstrated his genuine and profound concern for his fellow human beings and a willingness to make great personal sacrifice in the cause of science and human progress." That recommendation was from Max's new friend, Mayor Hubert Humphrey.

Max's talent for landing friends in high places was eventually more than a match for Vice Chairman John G. Jackson. The Committee on Character and Fitness relented, and Max was at last a lawyer. Max had every reason to believe that as soon as his hitch in the CPS was over, he would return to New York City and begin a successful career in law.

There was a piece of starvation folklore that Keys was eager to challenge during the experiment: that starvation somehow sharpened the senses. While he could believe that hungry people might somehow be more sensitive to the presence of food, with a heightened awareness of food sights and food smells, Keys found it difficult to believe that hunger actually improved hearing and seeing. He devised an elaborate series of tests to examine that possibility.

Keys was right about vision. He evaluated the sight of the men by measuring the smallest circles each could see in a constant level of light at a distance of fifteen feet. Starvation had no impact on their vision as the result stayed close to .69 millimeters for the duration of the experiment. Keys also tested the frequency at which successive light flashes appeared to fuse into an uninterrupted light source. That aspect of vision also did not improve with starvation, nor did it suffer.

The results of the hearing tests were more interesting. Keys marched the volunteers to a soundproof room within the headquarters of KUOM, the university's radio station. Using a Maico D-5 audiometer, Keys measured guinea pig hearing before, during, and after starvation. Keys found that hearing improved across the board, especially at the lower frequencies, where the results improved by a full standard deviation. Interviews with the men confirmed the results anecdotally: all the test subjects reported extremely low tolerance for loud music and speech.

Keys was at a loss to explain the result. He theorized that starvation had induced both lower production of earwax and a larger auditory canal, as the tissues of the ear shrunk away from their cartilage framework. In any case, an old wives' tale had been partially confirmed: hunger sharpened hearing.

Henry read and reread the letter, mailed in March but delivered in June, worn and frayed from its journey across a wartorn world. His parents were coming to Minneapolis. His father, Henry Caesar Scholberg, was retiring from the missionary life at the age of sixty-six. He was returning to Minnesota for good. The war forced his parents on a circuitous, nerve-wracking route home via Australia, across the Pacific, and finally making landfall in California. Then followed the long voyage into the heartland by rail. When the exhausted Scholbergs arrived in Minneapolis, they hadn't seen their son in six years. It was near the end of the starvation phase.

While his mother greeted other long lost family members and inventoried their luggage in town, Henry's father took a streetcar to the stadium alone. Henry greeted him at Gate 27.

He was shocked at his son's appearance, the pinched cheeks, the bony limbs. It was more than the lost weight. Henry had grown taller in the six years they had been separated. His eyes, too, were bright and knowing in an adult way. Henry's father was having the unusual experience of seeing his emaciated son as a man for the first time.

"Welcome to Unit 115," Henry said, shaking his dad's hand. He led him inside.

Inside the lab, Henry's father took a brief course from the staff on how to be a designated buddy, so that father and son could walk outside the stadium together without chaperone. The scientists instructed the elder Henry on how important it was for his son to eat nothing outside of Shevlin Hall. They conveyed to Henry's father how important Henry's data was, especially this late in the experiment, with a couple of men already gone. Henry's father was thus certified to act as his son's companion.

They had a lot to talk about. In the days leading up to the visit, Henry had wondered if he should be worried about a confrontation with his father over his pacifism, but he really wasn't. Maybe it was because he'd already been in the CPS for two years and it would seem a little ridiculous to fight about it now. Maybe it was because he was just so glad to see him. And, of course, there was always the possibility that he felt that way because hunger had made him irrational.

"How are you feeling?" his father asked. They were walking on a path along the Mississippi River, which was finally free of the chunks of ice that had dotted the shoreline through May. It was a walk Henry knew by heart, a well-worn path on his weekly journey of twenty-two miles. Seeing the river with his father made him aware of it in a different way, as he noticed the beauty of the cold water and the signs of the approaching spring. The route had been Henry's favorite before, but not because of the scenery. Henry loved the route because it took him by the Wonder bread factory, where he could swim in the smell of fresh bread baked on an industrial scale.

"How am I feeling?" said Henry. "As well as can be expected."

"Is it difficult?" asked his father.

Henry shrugged. "Some men have cheated. Some have gone nuts."

"But not you?"

"Well, I haven't cheated."

His father chuckled at that.

"I've been awful a couple of times," said Henry. "Said things in anger I really regret."

"Are you glad you volunteered?" his father asked.

Henry stopped walking and watched a giant log float slowly down the river. "I am, Dad. This thing has undressed us. The guys I thought would be strong—they've turned out to be weak. I thought I would take a beating—and I'm still sticking around."

"You seem stronger to me," said his father.

Henry was shocked, both because of the rare praise from his stern father and because the word "strong" was the last word he would use to describe himself at that moment.

Henry and his father both stared out at the river. "The hunger is just awful now in India," said Henry's father. "Even worse than when you were there. In Bengal they have no way of disposing of all the bodies. People are pouring into the cities from the country-side looking for food—it's just devastating."

There was a long silence. "If what you're doing here could help those people in some way . . . that would truly be the Lord's work."

They resumed walking. As Keys' tests had indicated, the intellective capacity of the men in the study was in large part unaffected by hunger, it just took more time for them to perform any given mental calculation. So they were a few miles down the road before Henry realized that his father may have just given his approval for what he was doing.

Keys had been steadily angling for press coverage of the experiment since before it started. He recognized that publicity would help secure future lab funding, and he was always well aware of the advantages of self-promotion. There had been coverage in the local papers, of course, but national press for conscientious objectors was harder to come by in a nation enthusiastically at war. That all changed on June 29 when the laboratory received a photographer from the most important magazine in the country: *Life*. They were going to do a photo essay about the experiment. For Keys, it was a public relations home run.

The photographer *Life* assigned was Wallace Kirkland. Kirkland had been a social worker before discovering photography. He had worked directly for the famous Jane Addams at Hull House, her pioneering mission for the urban poor in Chicago. Kirkland began photographing the boys of Hull House and the surrounding area. His renown as a photographer grew, and he was hired as a staff photographer by *Life* in 1936, the year of the magazine's founding. This would not be his first assignment to photograph the hungry. Kirkland traveled the world for *Life,* and he had been one of the only photographers allowed to photograph Gandhi at the 1940 All India Congress. Gandhi granted Kirkland an audience because of his association with Jane Addams, whom Gandhi greatly admired.

Even the worldly Kirkland was stunned as he was led through the laboratory. Skeletal young men with hollow stares drifted like ghosts through the catacombs beneath the stadium. Some were being measured by men in lab coats in various ways, their shirts off to better display their protruding ribs and hollow stomachs. The whole thing was hard to believe, especially that men would volunteer for this treatment. There were plenty of opportunities for intriguing photographs: A grown man licking his plate. A treasured stash of cookbooks. Henry Scholberg's edema-swollen leg.

There were also significant photographic challenges. Most of the windowless rooms of the lab were poorly lit. The quarters were cramped and it was hard to get far enough away to adequately frame the subjects. Kirkland took a picture of two shirtless men on treadmills from the back, their shoulder blades protruding. One young man was strapped to a menacing-looking table that rotated and tilted, with electrodes strapped to his chest and foot—Kirkland noted that the table was for testing blood circulation at various positions—"this is something like tests given fliers to determine resistance to blackout."

Kirkland wanted a photograph of Keys in the spread, and he could tell as Keys hovered in the background that the scientist did as well. He set up a posed shot of Keys, in his lab coat and tie, measuring the bare chest of James Plaugher with a giant caliper. Kirkland liked the contrast of the towering Plaugher being measured by the stocky Keys.

Kirkland also wanted to shoot a portrait of a volunteer outside the stadium, where the light was better and the background would be something other than the unending, unattractive concrete of the bowels of the stadium. He wanted one of the most gaunt volunteers to pose with his shirt off, someone who looked unnaturally thin, someone whose every rib would be on display. Kirkland didn't have the volunteer face the camera directly, he turned him slightly so that his ribs would cast shadows in the afternoon light. The subject he chose combed his hair neatly for the photograph—emaciated or not, everyone he knew read *Life*. He even tried to smile for Kirkland—he wanted to look triumphant, like a noble man taking a stand for his beliefs. The resulting smile looked tired, though, faraway and sad, as if the subject wanted to explain what true, consuming hunger felt like to the readers of *Life*, but knew it would be impossible. The subject of the photograph was Sam Legg.

Keys and Dr. Henry Longstreet Taylor were reviewing changes to individual diets in Keys' office on the evening of July 3, 1945. They had managed to postpone the hated task all day, so it was late, and they spoke quietly in the dark room. With any luck, it would be one of the last times they had to adjust diets, as the starvation phase neared its end. Taylor was smoking, something Keys disapproved of, but Keys was letting it slide. Deciding whose food to cut was the worst job the senior staff had, and it got harder each week. The once faceless subject numbers all had names for them now. Keys and Taylor dreaded looking at those faces after slashing their already meager ration of bread and potatoes. If smoking a Lucky Strike somehow made it easier for Taylor to make those decisions with him, then Keys was willing to let it pass.

"Number 108?" said Keys. "Haven't we already cut his diet?"

Taylor nodded. "That's Lester Glick. He's been stuck at 121 pounds for two weeks."

"Couldn't that be edema?"

"Could be," said Taylor. "We've taken that into account. Still, no weight loss for two weeks—zero. He's supposed to end up at 114 pounds. We have to cut his food."

Keys sighed. "Okay—how much do you want to cut?"

Taylor hesitated. "Two slices of bread and 20 grams of potatoes."

"My god," said Keys. It was a devastating cut in calories. "Go ahead, go ahead."

Taylor made an annotation on Glick's file as Keys rubbed his temples. "Tomorrow's the Fourth of July," said Keys. "Are we doing anything special for the men?"

Taylor shrugged. "Nothing planned."

"Is there any extra food we can give them?"

"I guess that's up to you," said Taylor. "We can't exactly give them hot dogs and cheeseburgers." He thought for a moment. "I suppose we could give them a dish of watermelon balls without endangering the data."

"Do it," said Keys.

"Okay," said Taylor. He made a note, and opened the file of the next subject up for a reduction in bread and potatoes. He handed it to Keys. "Subject Number 130," he said. He pulled another cigarette from his pack.

The new individual menus were posted on the bulletin board the next morning. James Graham saw that Lester Glick's ration had been cut yet again, and he knew that his friend would be despondent. Even by guinea pig standards, Lester passionately loved food. He had been one of the few volunteers visibly, although not excessively, overweight when the study began. Lester could spend long hours talking about the hearty fare his mother put on the table of their Mennonite farmhouse in Sugar Creek, Ohio: fried pork tenderloin, fried rabbit, fried mush, pudding meat, and hard-boiled eggs pickled in red beet juice. One favorite treat back in Sugar Creek was two quarts of strawberries mixed with half a loaf of broken bread and a gallon of fresh milk. Graham knew that Glick felt he was being unfairly punished for his edema, and would take the news about his latest food reduction hard.

Graham found Glick sitting on the end of his bed. One look confirmed that Glick already knew.

"Let's go into town," Graham suggested.

"No thanks," mumbled Glick.

"Come on, we'll go to that diner on Fifth, drink coffee, watch people eat lunch—it'll be fun!" It was an activity they had enjoyed several times in the past.

"No thanks," said Glick again.

"Lester, I won't take no for an answer. We need to go out." Graham had always been a rock of stability, one of the few men in the lab who still had energy enough to look out for someone other than himself. Glick knew he couldn't resist.

"All right," said Glick, "I'll go with you—but only if you're buying the coffee."

Graham laughed. "You're on," he said.

At the restaurant, the two ordered their black coffees and settled back to observe what the people of Minneapolis were eating. Their attention soon focused on a well-dressed lady who had ordered the pork chop dinner, one of their favorite meals to watch. The two guinea pigs were horrified when she ate only about half of the meat. She then pushed aside the nuts and bacon that garnished her string beans as if it were mere decoration. Finally, she ate only half of her salad, leaving behind the mouthwatering radishes and carrots.

Glick lost himself in a vivid fantasy about eating all the food that remained on her plate and wiping it clean with a piece of bread. "I can't believe how much food she's wasting," he said. When Jim didn't reply, he looked over. Graham was absolutely fuming, glaring furiously at the wasteful diner. Glick chuckled . . . Graham had suggested the trip to take their minds off the experiment.

The lady ordered dessert: coconut cream pie. Jim and Lester Glick both stared, open mouthed, as the waiter carried the towering slice by their table. It almost entirely obscured its plate.

"That," whispered Jim, "is God's prize creation."

The lady proceeded to push the whipped cream off the top. She then nibbled daintily at the filling, leaving most of it, and the delicious, flaky crust, untouched. She paid her bill and left the restaurant.

Before Lester could comment on what had happened, he realized that Jim had left their table. In fact, he had followed the lady onto the street in a rage. By the time Lester caught up, James Graham was waving his bony arms and ranting like a lunatic.

"Do you have any idea how much food you just wasted?" he yelled. "Do you have any idea how much hunger is in the world—hunger that you are contributing to?"

The lady was shocked by the behavior of the exceedingly skinny, exceedingly nervy young man who was lecturing her. "You're . . . you're some kind of crazy man!" she said. She bolted down the street.

Lester started laughing. "You were right Jim," he said. "That was fun." Glick laughed so hard that he forgot his reduction in

bread, the months remaining in the experiment, and even the nag-
ging pain in his chest that wouldn't seem to go away.

July 28, 1945, was a day Sam Legg had been anticipating since
the beginning of the experiment—the last day of the starvation
phase. He had been telling himself as his body weakened and his
thoughts grew darker that the day was soon approaching when
his gnawing hunger would finally be satisfied. Slowly, the long,
dark Minnesota winter gave way to spring, and then to summer—and then it was here. The end of July, the end of the starvation phase. Legg was too tired to be jubilant. But he was relieved.
He was almost to the finish line.

While many of the men had seen their weight losses slow or
stop due to edema, Legg's weight had actually plummeted, due to
a bout of excessive diuresis, urination even more extreme than the
polyuria now typical in the other men. Legg's weight was actually
well below his predictive curve: the 5 foot 10 inch Sam Legg
weighed only 105.6 pounds, down from his original weight of
142.

The anticipation of July 28 became mingled with dread when
he learned that he was scheduled to take the Harvard Fitness Test
on that same day. It was an appropriate milestone for his last day
in the nightmare of hunger. He began worrying about the test
days in advance. He was too weak even to climb the stairs to their
barracks without taking breaks; he couldn't contemplate keeping
up with the racing treadmill. He wrote a sonnet in his journal to
express his dread:

> No man can ever equal the machine;
> No sinew, bone and muscle can compete
> Against the monster. In the clash between
> the two, we men must always meet defeat.

His temper had flared at dinner the night before. The man ahead of him in line at Shevlin Hall told the server that the crust of burnt macaroni clinging to the edge of the pan should be a part of his portion. Legg had been eyeing that chunk his whole time in line.

"No, that should be mine," he said.

"Give it to me," said the man in front of him.

"Go to hell," said Legg, shoving him with his bony shoulder.

They both quickly dropped their precious trays and began hitting each other. With their thin arms and their weak, uncoordinated punches, they looked like two fighting marionettes. Even so, a few good punches landed before the rest of the pacifists in line could tear them apart.

The scientists and technicians were waiting for Legg at the treadmill the next morning. Now in the last week of the starvation phase, they were attaching safety straps to the men, so rapid was their collapse and so weak were their bodies. Legg paused at the foot of the treadmill, as if contemplating not getting on. The scientists looked at each other, wondering what they might do if a subject refused to do the test. After what they had witnessed for the last nine months, they could certainly sympathize.

Legg climbed onto the treadmill, and held his arms out as they attached the safety straps around his narrow waist.

"Ready?" said the technician. Legg gave a tired nod. The tech flipped the switch and Legg began his twenty-minute walk at 3.5 miles per hour, at a 20 percent grade.

The walk portion didn't seem eternal to just Legg, it seemed to take forever to the anxious technicians as well. While all the volunteers were still walking the mandatory twenty-two miles a week, Legg's pace had slowed to a crawl in the final weeks of starvation, well below the treadmill's 3.5 miles per hour. The technicians could tell the wheezing subject was struggling to keep up, and they dreaded accelerating the belt as he exhausted himself during the preliminary walking phase. Legg looked so bony and weak. It was just impossible to imagine this tired creature running on the treadmill at full speed.

"Ready?" asked the tech again, as the twenty-minute walk concluded. Legg gave a sad nod from the treadmill without looking down. A dial was turned, and the treadmill doubled in speed.

He collapsed in nineteen seconds. It happened so quickly that the technicians took a moment to grab him. For that second, Legg dangled above the speeding treadmill supported by just the safety straps. The staff quickly got him down and laid him out on a cot where they could complete their measurements. His score was an abysmal 6, down from a 72 in control, and a 32 at S12. Overall, it represented a 91 percent drop in his fitness. His deterioration was far worse than the average drop of 72 percent.

The crying started as the men were taking his pulse. Without knowing how to comfort him, they tried to complete their measurements quickly. It was an era when the sight of a man crying was still rare and terrible. They might have told him that his collapse was not unusual and nothing to be ashamed of, although only one man would do worse on the final fitness test. They might have told him that his collapse was understandable in light of his greater than average weight loss. In the end, they just hurriedly completed their measurements and left the crying man alone as soon as possible. His sobs grew into wails as the men departed. All felt guilty for the culpability they had in the collapse of Sam Legg.

In his diary that night, Legg wrote about his last day in semi-starvation: *I have never been so ashamed of any performance as I was then, but had completely let go of myself and couldn't do anything but go on sobbing . . . ever since I've felt like a quitter and I hate quitters.*

Later that evening, Bob Willoughby was summoned to Dr. Keys' office. Everyone in the barracks knew that Plaugher had been called in earlier, and had been gone for over an hour. Willoughby expected more of the usual veiled accusations when he wearily walked into the office.

"Sit down, Bob," said Dr. Keys. Dr. Taylor was standing to his left. "I want to ask you again if you've cheated."

Willoughby was startled. The question was usually not put to them that directly. "No—of course not," he said. Keys pushed a piece of graph paper across his desk.

"Take a look at this for me," he said. It was a smooth curve, with points plotted against it in neat, scientific sharp pencil. Willoughby knew his predictive graph well, but Keys went on to explain it anyway

"Right now you weigh 136.4 pounds. Twelve weeks ago, you weighed 137.72 pounds. Your total weight loss in twenty-four weeks has been only 18 percent."

Willoughby fumed, but remained silent. Keys continued.

"The average, as you might know, has been about a twenty-four percent loss. Yet you, despite being on one of the most restricted diets, don't approach that loss."

Keys sat back and waited for Willoughby to respond.

"I didn't cheat," said Willoughby.

"I think you did," said Keys. "And I think you'll feel better about it if you face the issue squarely."

It was too much for Willoughby. "Jim and I are just big guys!" he shouted. "Maybe it's because we're more athletic than anyone else here, did you think of that? We're the two fittest, strongest guys here, and you think we're both cheating? Do you think that's a coincidence?"

Taylor and Keys looked at each other. With a measure of sympathy in his voice, Taylor spoke up. "Actually, Bob, James Plaugher did cheat. He's been cheating since the beginning."

"A bread crust!" said Willoughby. "He told you guys all about that."

"I'm afraid it's worse than that," said the scientist. "He confessed everything. He ate a whole sandwich he found on the ground, he stole a student's lunch and ate it, and he's even been eating garbage routinely. He told us all about it. We know you two were close friends—we think you probably did it together."

Willoughby was stunned. He couldn't believe his friend cheated. He couldn't believe Jim had lied to him. He realized how guilty this made him look, as if he and Jim had become friends only to help each other undermine the buddy system and eat off the diet. His shock turned to anger as he thought of the hunger and pain he had endured for months, only to be convicted of cheating without a trial. He stood up. "I don't care what Jim did, I don't care what you think, and I don't care what your graph says—I DID NOT CHEAT." He stormed out of the room.

Keys was not convinced. Plaugher was dropped from the experiment, and he checked himself into the psychiatric ward of the university hospital—the second test subject to find a home there. Keys expressed his characteristic distaste for the men too weak to complete the experiment in his review of the Plaugher case: "In summary, this subject's latent personality weaknesses were amplified and brought to the surface by the stress. He did not have the strength to carry out the program or the capacity to decide unequivocally to get out of the unpleasant situation. Thus he developed an experimentally induced neurosis characterized by such symptoms as indecisiveness, self-deprecation, feelings of guilt, restlessness, nervous tension, compulsive gum chewing, and eating off diet."

Willoughby remained at the lab, but Keys, convinced he was a cheater, did not use his data in the final study. Without a confession or definite proof, Keys called Willoughby's crime a "probable breaking of the diet," indicated by "indirect but convincing evidence." That evidence consisted mainly of Willoughby's failure to lose weight as predicted and his friendship with Plaugher. Keys also said that the indications of neurosis in Willoughby's MMPI were more significant than anything found in interviews or his diary because Willoughby was so "hopelessly unable to express himself."

The thirty-two men who made it to the rehabilitation phase were in many ways different than the men who had shown up at Memorial Stadium in November of 1944. They were smaller— they had dropped from an average of 152.7 pounds to 115.6 pounds, an average weight loss of 24.29 percent. They were shorter, too—the average man had lost about a third of a centimeter in height. Their total blood volume had been reduced by almost 500 cubic centimeters. The heart that pumped that blood had shrunk by 17 percent. More significant, and more difficult for Keys to measure, their world had shrunk. The men had come to Minnesota to be part of a global mission to help all of humanity. Now they didn't care about starving refugees, or VE day, or self-government inside CPS Unit 115. Now their world consisted only of the South Tower of Memorial Stadium and the food line at Shevlin Hall.

One of the ways Brozek came up with to evaluate the overall deterioration of the men was ingenious in its simplicity. Who knew better than the men themselves? He had the guinea pigs periodically rate each other on a scale from zero to five, with zero being normal and five being extreme deterioration. The average score at S24 was 2.3. At S24, the test subjects evaluated Subject Number 109 as the man among them showing the least deterioration, with a low score of 1.1—it was Phillip Liljengren, who also happened to be the oldest guinea pig at thirty-three. The man whom they evaluated as most deteriorated, with a score of 3.7, was Henry Scholberg.

Sam Legg walked back to the stadium from Shevlin Hall after their last meal of the starvation phase. He was close enough to the group of test subjects in front of him to be in compliance with the buddy system. He was far enough behind them to enjoy the illusion of solitude. The campus was relatively empty for summer. The sight of the streets without snow or ice still surprised him after the long winter. Once again he walked by the fraternity houses on University Avenue seized by the navy to house their officer candidates. He walked by the university's ancient armory, whose castlelike turrets seemed more suited to the training of crusading knights than soldiers for Eisenhower. Finally, he walked through Gate 27 and up the stairs for what he knew would be his last night in starvation, his last night too cold, too tired to turn in bed, too hungry to think or dream of anything but food. He had been counting on this day for six months. Whatever weak sense of victory he might have had was killed earlier by his humiliating collapse on the treadmill. As he returned to the barracks, he thought about enduring another night without food. Most of the men were giddy about the advent of rehabilitation. Sam Legg couldn't think any further ahead than the long hungry night. The anticipation of it filled him with pure panic.

CHAPTER SEVEN

◄◦►

RESTRICTED REHABILITATION

MAX KAMPELMAN FID-
GETED with the other vol-
unteers in the line at the
door to Shevlin Hall. It was Sunday morning, July 29—the first
day of rehabilitation. They were ravenous, as usual, in the final
excruciating minutes before breakfast. The fifteen-hour span
between dinner and breakfast was the longest interval they went
without eating, making the morning line one of the tensest events
of the day. There was an excited buzz through the line that day as
the men contemplated what might be served. Memories of the
May 26 relief meal with its gravy and jelly hung heavily over
the group. Some men thought they smelled bacon through the
thick oak door. Some swore they could hear eggs being broken
over a sizzling skillet, and orange juice being poured into tall
glasses.

Max had tried hard to avoid being swept up in the optimism
that flooded the laboratory in the days leading up to R1. He
noted to the others that the scientists carefully referred to the new
phase as "restricted" rehabilitation. No one else seemed to be
worried by that qualifier. In the line that morning, it was difficult
even for Max to avoid the general feeling that the worst was over.
There was a collective feeling of accomplishment: they had made
it through starvation. And this breakfast would be their reward.
When the doors to the serving line swung open, it was all Max
could do to contain a shout of celebration.

163

He grabbed his tray and waited his turn. When he got to the servers, he watched stunned as the dietician looked at his chart, carefully weighed out a scoop of unflavored farina, and plopped it in his tray, just as he had done each of the previous 168 days. The food hadn't changed. Max had to stop himself from asking if there had been some mistake. The excited chatter in the line stopped one man at a time as each guinea pig filed through and received his disappointing, wholly unsatisfying allotment.

Henry Scholberg could sense the disappointment in his peers as they sat down with their trays in stunned silence. He did not share it. Henry didn't know then that his peers had evaluated him as the most deteriorated at S24, but it would not have surprised him. He might have evaluated himself that way. He knew he had blown up more times, acted more irritably, and refined his technique with profanity more than anyone else in the experiment. But as he watched the men take their places with their inadequately filled trays, he felt a sense of contentment he had never felt before.

Sure, he hadn't always acted perfectly. There were occasions, as when he humiliated George Ebeling, that he would regret all his life. But he had made it. He was one of just thirty-six men to make it into the experiment, and he was one of only thirty-two to complete it. Unlike many of the sharp, confident volunteers, Henry had never been certain that he would get through the experiment, even on Day 1. But he had made it. As Henry savored his delicious, steaming 200 grams of farina, he had never felt more proud.

While the food was the same over the next few days, they were supposedly getting more of it. It was hard to tell, as the servers at Shevlin continued to scoop out twice a day carefully measured quantities of the familiar turnips, cabbage, and macaroni. Over the next few days, the guinea pigs heard that they had been secretly divided into four subgroups of eight men, each receiving either 400, 800, 1,200, or 1,600 more calories than they had in starvation. Some received a protein supplement. Some received a vitamin supplement. No one was supposed to know what group he was in, so they tried to figure it out on their own by observing the food on everyone else's plate. None of the hungry men believed he was in the highest caloric group. Most felt like they were in the lowest.

For those men actually in the lower groups, the disappointment of rehabilitation was crushing. Four hundred additional calories amounted to little more than a few slices of whole wheat bread a day. They still had to walk twenty-two miles a week; they still had to go everywhere with a buddy. The temptation to cheat was as strong as ever, as was the depression, the fatigue, and the physical discomfort. After six months of hunger, the men had prayed that July 29 would bring relief. It did not.

In a development that surprised everyone, many of the men began to lose weight even more rapidly early in the recovery period. The scientists ascertained that the weight loss was caused by the reduction of edema as the body healed; the body was shedding heavy fluid weight faster than it could regenerate healthy flesh. It was, in other words, a sign of recovery. The scientists found it fascinating. Most of the men, however, already down on average to 115.6 pounds, found it impossible to take pleasure in further weight loss.

On August 6, Max was passing by the laundry after a tiring three-mile walk to start the second week of rehabilitation. He noticed a crowd gathered around Bob Villwock's radio, a crowd listening to the news with unusual intensity. The war had been lurching across the Pacific since VE day, but few of them still in the experiment could muster much concern anymore. To most of the guinea pigs, it seemed like the war and the experiment had both been going on forever, and would last forever. Max walked into the room to see what had caused the men to abandon their apathy.

A new kind of bomb had leveled a Japanese city called Hiroshima. It was apparently "an important Japanese Army base," although Max had never heard of it before it was destroyed. Max listened to the broadcast carefully, but details were sketchy. The only thing that was clear was that something very important had happened in the war.

Only a few more details were available in the evening paper, but at least the new weapon was given a name. ATOMIC BOMB HITTING JAPS, TRUMAN REVEALS. Truman described the weapon in apocalyptic terms in his statement to the American people: "It is an atomic bomb. It is a harnessing of the basic power of the universe. The force from which the sun draws its power has been loosed against those who brought war to the Far East."

Max pored over the story in the barracks, memorizing the superlatives that the reporters seemed to have exhausted themselves producing. The bomb was 2,000 times heavier than the biggest bomb used in the war. Sixty-five thousand people had somehow managed to work secretly in two locations to manufacture it. An astonishing two billion dollars had been spent to develop it. The Japanese, for their part, refused to believe that such destruction could be caused by a single bomb.

Over the next two days, Max learned more details. A *Star Journal* headline reported ALL LIVING THINGS SEARED TO DEATH. Unofficial American sources estimated the Japanese dead at 100,000. Max inhaled the stories, horrified but fascinated by humanity's newest weapon. A picture of Hiroshima began to take shape in Max's mind, a picture of charred bodies and vast ruin. A change began taking place in Max, a change as significant as anything that took place in the experiment, but one that would have been impossible for even Keys to quantify.

For many men, news of the atom bomb might have confirmed the wisdom of pacifism—man's destructive capacity had grown too great for war to be a reasonable option. For Max, though, the horrible details of Hiroshima had the opposite effect. The push of a single button could now obliterate millions of lives. The atomic bomb had changed the world in a fundamental way. Max had no doubt that other nations would soon harness this mysterious and terrible power. Max's belief that the "power of love" could be a match for the armies of the world now seemed tragically naïve. Passive resistance in the face of the "basic power of the universe" was futile. Allowing evil men to use such weapons when the use of violence might stop them—that would be immoral.

It was a hot summer day in Minnesota, a day that Max spent surrounded, as he had been for two years, by other conscientious objectors. Max had joined the CPS as an idealistic young pacifist on June 1, 1943. His idealism had survived a tour at an unproductive conservation camp, a school for mentally ill children, and six months of starvation. His idealism had been rocked by the increasingly horrific disclosures of the Nazi crimes against the Jewish people, yet it had survived. But on the day the U.S. dropped the atomic bomb on Hiroshima, Max Kampelman stopped being a pacifist.

Three days after Hiroshima, the U.S. dropped a second, more powerful atomic bomb on Nagasaki. On August 15, Emperor Hirohito went on the radio to explain the unexplainable to his people. "The war situation has developed not necessarily to Japan's advantage . . . Moreover the enemy has begun to employ a new and most cruel bomb, the power of which to do damage is indeed incalculable, taking toll of many innocent lives. Should we continue to fight, it would not only result in the ultimate collapse and obliteration of the Japanese nation, but also it would lead to the extinction of human civilization."

The war was over. In the August 15 *Star Journal*, news of the Japanese capitulation shared the front page with word that the rationing of canned food in the United States had ended.

Nine and a half weeks remained in the experiment.

Sam Legg looked in the mirror. It was R3, the third week of rehabilitation. He had taken a hot shower in preparation for his evening out. All the men had learned to savor long, hot showers, one of the only times they could really feel completely warm. That brief physical pleasure evaporated as he leaned forward with two hands on the sink, a towel around his waist, to stare at his reflection and inventory his physical deterioration.

His once wavy hair was coarse and thin. He knew it would fall out in clumps as he combed it. His sallow skin was dry and cold. Around his eyes, in a spectacle pattern, were distinct patches of darkened skin. These dark patches around the eyes, unexplainable by the doctors, were present in nineteen of the men. Sam's lips and his fingernails were blue, another common condition unexplainable by the doctors. He once overheard Dr. Keys say that it was reminiscent of the cyanosis he had seen on mountaintops. Some hair follicles on Sam's upper arms had hardened, giving his skin the texture of a nutmeg grater. The scientists called that follicular hyperkeratosis. On other parts of his body, he had permanent gooseflesh. His homely body was defined by sharp angles, bumps, and points as his bones poked against their shrinking cage of flesh.

To Sam, as he studied himself, his eyes were the most striking change. They were not bloodshot, as might be expected in a man as profoundly tired as Sam. In contrast, the corneas were unnaturally white. The lack of redness, what the doctors called "avascularity," was noticeable in all the men, even from a distance. The condition was so puzzling to the scientists that they tried to induce redness in some of their eyes with a mild soap solution, but could not. Sam's lifeless corneas were the color of unglazed white porcelain. He tried to will himself to smile as he stared down his reflection. He was getting a visit from his sister that night, and he needed to assure himself that he could at least do a passable imitation of a man getting by. But he wasn't. Sam was a slave to his hunger. Day and night his flesh cried for nutrition, his animal needs triumphing over any higher purpose he might once have felt. While it seemed like every guinea pig thought he was in the lowest of the four caloric groups, Sam *knew* he was.

Even the thought of leaving the stadium for a few hours with his sister offered him no pleasure. While his sister ate dinner with their friends, Sam Legg, Subject No. 20, would have to go outside until the meal was over, and pass the time by chopping wood.

Keys was on his way home to Lake Owasso when the hospital telephoned. His wife, Margaret, had to give him the message as he stepped out of his car in the driveway. One of the volunteers, Samuel Legg, had chopped off the fingers of his left hand—that was all she knew. Keys walked inside to sit on the couch for a moment and absorb the news before getting back in his car for the long trip back to Minneapolis.

"Maybe it was an accident," said Margaret, trying to be comforting.

"Maybe," he said. "But I doubt it. The same man had an accident last week, dropped his car on the same hand."

There was a brief silence.

"My god, Margaret," he said. "I am torturing them."

In the hospital, Keys walked briskly up to the room. Legg was in the regular ward, not the psychiatric ward, the doctors on duty having apparently believed the incident was an accident and not self-mutilation. Legg was asleep when Keys walked in. His emaciated body looked tiny on the hospital bed; his size also made the bulging bandage on his left hand look huge. Some blood had managed to soak through the thick layers of gauze, forming a row of three small dark red circles. Keys walked quietly to the foot of the bed, picked up the chart, and read the terse medical description of the young man who had been in his care. Twenty-nine years old. Had chopped off the three middle fingers of his left hand with an ax. Condition was stable.

Sam Legg had been in trouble, and Keys had missed it. He cursed himself for not removing the man after his "accident" with the car the week before. The problem was, many of the men were deteriorating just as badly. Legg's decline, while significant, was not unusual. According to the deterioration ratings the men gave themselves, no fewer than seven men were holding up worse than Legg at S24: Henry Scholberg, George Ebeling, Marshall Sutton, William Anderson, Carlyle Frederick, James Graham, and Lester Glick. How could he have removed Legg without also removing them? And how could he dismiss eight out of thirty-two remaining men without destroying the experiment? He couldn't. Keys looked at Legg's hand, hidden behind the bandage, forever maimed. Maybe that was the lesson, thought Keys, maybe they shouldn't have conducted the experiment at all. Maybe the scientific goals he set were not possible to achieve in a humane way. Keys tried to bury his doubt and his guilt in a study of the cold, clinical details of Sam's medical chart. He sighed as he placed the file back in its holder at the foot of the bed.

Legg stirred, and opened his eyes. Keys could tell by the glassy expression that he was heavily medicated.

"Hello, Sam," he said. Legg blinked twice.

"Doctor Keys?" he said. His voice was scratchy. Keys handed him a glass of water from the tray near his bedside. Legg gulped loudly and handed the glass back to Keys. A heavy silence came over the room. Keys heard the squeaking of a gurney rolling by, the hushed laughter of the nurses at the end of the hall, a radio playing the Andrews Sisters somewhere far away. Everywhere, since VJ day, were the sounds of celebration. Everywhere except the laboratory. Keys realized Sam was still awake and watching him. The doctor gathered his composure.

"Is there anything I can do for you, Sam?" asked Dr. Keys.

"Yes," said Sam.

Keys leaned closer to hear.

"Keep me in the experiment," he said.

Keys straightened. "Why . . . why would you want to?"

"Please," said Sam. "Keep me in. For the hungry." The answer was as sterile as the air of the hospital room, satisfying neither of them.

"Sam, I am afraid I can't keep you in," said Keys. "You need rest and decent meals. You've done a fine job, but I just don't see how I can keep you in the experiment after this. And what's more, I don't see why you would want to."

Sam realized he was on the verge of being kicked out of the experiment, his data erased as though he had never been to Minneapolis at all, like Watkins, Weygandt, Willoughby, and Plaugher. He could almost feel his work evaporating, the blood samples, the psychological interviews, the sperm samples, the dreaded Harvard Fitness Tests. The hunger and the medication made the words bunch up in his throat, made his eyes heavy. Sam willed himself into wakefulness. His chance was slipping away—Sam knew he needed to explain at that moment to Dr. Keys why he *had* to stay in the experiment.

"Doctor," he said, his voice still hoarse and quiet, "for the rest of my life, people are going to ask me what I did during the war. This experiment is my chance to give an honorable answer to that question."

The conversation and the medication had exhausted him. He drifted off to sleep, leaving Keys alone with his thoughts.

The news about Sam ran through the barracks as though a third atomic bomb had been dropped. They all regarded Sam as an almost fatherly presence, patiently shepherding them through the CPS just as he had guided them through French grammar. He had been one of the most educated, most impressive subjects. He had also been one of the most experienced, veterans of the CPS, having been inducted four months before Pearl Harbor. Only Lester Glick had been in longer. Sam was one of their leaders, and he had cracked up. If it could happen to Sam Legg, it could happen to any of them.

Every man remaining in the experiment understood Sam's despair in rehabilitation. The disappointment had flattened them all. Two by two they visited Sam in the hospital, incorporating that walk into their twenty-two miles for the week. All were surprised that Dr. Keys had kept him in the experiment. Sam's rehabilitation meals were brought to him in the hospital in the kind of white cardboard containers used by Chinese restaurants.

Sam's happiness at being kept in was much easier for them to understand. No one wanted to have come so far, only to see his contribution excised from the experiment. These young men were convinced that they were on the verge of the greatest accomplishment of their lives. The prospect of removal was devastating. Sam's decision to stay, and Keys' decision to allow it, cheered them all. Sam returned to the stadium after five days in the university hospital.

Keys was worried. For months it had seemed like the war would crawl to a close, one trench, one volcanic island at a time. Now, in an atomic flash, it was over. The rapidity of events was stunning. The war in Europe had been over since May 8. Relief workers were traveling to Europe by the shipload, without data from his laboratory. Every doctor in the world, it seemed, had a pet theory about what combination of vitamins could best heal the famished, what percentage of protein could speed recovery, and whether or not to skip normal feeding altogether in order to feed the weak intravenously and with stomach tubes. These were some of the very issues Keys had set out to address when he first proposed the study. In 1944, it had seemed that this was the exact moment in history to run the starvation experiment—a confluence of hunger on an unprecedented scale and the availability of willing guinea pigs. Now Keys feared that history might pass him by.

He knew it would be months, maybe even years, before the mountain of data they had accumulated could be assembled into a full-scale report. Even so, he hoped to throw something useful together for relief workers immediately, something he could perhaps even publish before the end of rehabilitation. Keys worked feverishly to assemble an interim report that would be of some practical use.

The problem was that Keys could not, as a man of science, offer conclusions before the experiment had finished, even though some important theories were already taking shape. The protein and vitamin supplements were one frustrating example. It appeared that neither the protein supplement nor the vitamin supplement had any appreciable effect on recovery. The "hexa-vitamin" given to half the men contained between one half and one full recommended daily allowance of vitamins A, C, D, riboflavin, niacin, and thiamine. The protein supplement given to half the men contained twenty grams of casein and soybean protein. To evaluate recovery, Keys tracked a range of data points from each man, including weight, body fat, pulse rate, and the depression score from the MMPI. Neither the vitamin nor the protein had any noticeable effect on any aspect of recovery. On the other hand, the four caloric groups recovered at rates almost exactly proportional to the number of calories they were receiving. Keys wanted to tell relief workers that they shouldn't trouble themselves preparing special protein feedings. Nor should they expect some miraculous vitamin formula to become an acceptable substitute for more food. He just couldn't bring himself to publish that information with the data from only four weeks of recovery.

Keys was working on the interim report late one night when Josef Brozek entered his office with a light knock.

"Hello, Yashka," said Keys.

Brozek nodded politely and sat in the chair in front of Keys' desk. "I bring a message from the natives," he said, in his thick Czech accent. He handed Keys a piece of paper.

It was a manifesto, of sorts, carefully written in the left-wing argot favored by so many of the subjects. The paper demanded, after a lengthy preamble about freedom of choice and the rights of man, that the buddy system be abolished.

Keys looked over his reading glasses at his colleague. "Of course we can't do this," he said.

Brozek nodded. "I know," he said.

"So why are you smiling?" asked Keys gruffly.

Brozek leaned forward in his chair. "It is a good sign, yes? The men are getting feisty."

Keys grunted as he digested Brozek's insight. "Well, nonetheless, we can't get rid of the buddy system now. And we certainly can't have the inmates thinking they can run the asylum. Call for a group meeting tomorrow after dinner."

The next evening, on August 29, 1945, halfway through the fifth week of rehabilitation, Keys stood before the thirty-two remaining men of the experiment. Legg was there with his bandaged hand. They made brief eye contact as Keys waited for the corps of volunteers to assemble.

"I know many of you feel the buddy system is burdensome," he said when they had all shuffled in. "I agree that it is. I want you all to know that I also feel it is still absolutely necessary. I appreciate your feelings very much, but the experiment goes only another seven weeks, and the buddy system will be with us until that final day. For seven weeks, we must all be ruled by scientific necessity, and not by our own individual wants and needs."

Keeping in mind what Brozek had said about rising feistiness, Keys scanned the group for signs of dissent. He found himself almost hoping for some kind of protest. They still looked tired and emaciated, but there did seem to be a little more life in their eyes than there had been at S24. Keys thought he even saw a few flashes of anger as he made his announcement, and that rise in energy pleased him greatly. Still, no one raised his voice to disagree with him.

"That is all," Keys said. And he walked out of the lab.

While Keys was thrilled that the men seemed to be coming back to life before his eyes, he was worried about the slow pace of the physical recovery. The men in the lower two caloric groups were barely gaining weight at all, although at least the weight loss appeared to have stopped as edema disappeared. After six weeks of rehabilitation, the men in the lowest caloric group had regained a miserable one tenth of one pound. Even the men receiving the highest caloric diet, almost double their diet in starvation, had regained only 6.5 pounds, less than one fifth of their total weight loss. It was one of the conclusions Keys was itching to share with relief workers, that it would take more than three thousand calories a day to facilitate recovery. It was yet another conclusion Keys couldn't share until the study was complete.

In general, all the indices of recovery followed the same sluggish pace as weight gain. The percentage of body fat was an exception. Fat, the body's emergency energy supply, had dropped more dramatically than body weight during starvation, and in recovery, body fat increased slightly faster. Pulse rates in the first six weeks of recovery had gone up on average only 4.2 beats per minute. They had dropped 17.9 beats per minute from 55.2 in control to 37.3 at S24 in one of the experiment's most striking changes. In two of the men, Roscoe Hinkle and Kenneth Tuttle, pulse rates actually continued to drop through the first six weeks of rehabilitation. All the men were depressed about the pace of their progress, and Keys didn't blame them. Keys wondered if they would get the chance to study recovery at all by adhering to the experiment's original design. Late one night, alone in his office with an array of downward sloping graphs arranged on his desk, he began to contemplate the unthinkable—drastically increasing the amount of food. He brought it up during the next day's meeting of the senior staff.

"You want to deviate from the plan?" asked Dr. Taylor. They had spent months designing the experiment, and Keys was usually the last among them to advocate improvisation, especially if that improvisation might be interpreted as some kind of unscientific compassion.

"Look, gentlemen," said Keys, sensing their surprise. "We're supposed to be learning about rehabilitation. Right now, we're not rehabilitating anyone. We've only got a few more weeks to study this group of men. I am afraid at this pace, we won't have seen any recovery at all." The men nodded in agreement. They all relished the thought of giving the men more food. As scientists, however, they needed to be convinced that it would not undermine the research.

"The point of this experiment," Keys continued, "was not to learn how to starve people—we brought these men here to learn how to rehabilitate people. All of us, especially the guinea pigs, have labored to create a pool of starved men to rehabilitate. I am satisfied that in the past five weeks we have proven that 400, 800, 1,200, and 1,600 additional calories won't do the job. We have a scientific duty in our remaining time to find out what will. Are we all in agreement?"

They all nodded. "Good," said Keys. "I'll announce it tomorrow."

The next day was September 9, 1945, a Sunday. The men were having another "relief meal," like the one they had had to mark the halfway point of the experiment. They again gorged themselves on starchy, homegrown favorites covered in gravy and served with rolls. Again, there was a general rise in spirits and conversation as the meal progressed and the men experienced full stomachs and a varied menu for the first time in months.

The cheerful chatter stopped cold when Keys stood to address them. A speech from Keys usually meant that someone had been thrown out of the lab or a group request was about to be denied. The men quietly scanned the room to see if anyone was missing.

"I am afraid that our study of rehabilitation has not been as efficient as I had hoped," Keys said somberly. "In order to boost our effectiveness, we are going to increase the food allotted to all four groups. Each group will increase by an average of 800 calories, meaning you will be consuming 1,200, 1,600, 2,000, or 2,400 more calories than you did in the starvation phase. Are there any questions?" In the absence of any response, Keys sat back down and resumed reviewing the high stack of notes he was editing for his interim report.

There was stunned silence as the men took it all in. After a six-week delay, they were finally going to get the rehabilitation phase they had all been waiting for.

The increased amount of food allowed them to shift to three meals a day, starting with a breakfast at 7:30. Sweet potatoes were added to the menu, as were real butter and jam. Immediately weights slowly rose, but spirits soared, as a gnawing desire for food stopped being each man's only companion. Just two days after the increase in meals, Brozek brought Keys another typed manifesto from the men.

Keys read it at his desk, trying to ignore the huge smile on his staff psychologist's face. The note had more signatures this time and was even more inflamed with left-wing bombast about strikes and non-cooperation. The men were insisting that the buddy system be abolished.

"What do you make of this?" Keys asked.

Brozek shrugged. "We are feeding them enough now, I wonder if we really need the buddy system any more. Plus, the men we have left—they are pretty tough. I don't know if you need to worry about them cheating so much. And . . . "

"What?" Keys interrupted.

"I am afraid, doctor, that if you do not give in on this, you may have to put down a general rebellion."

"And once again, you seem to find this insubordination amusing," said Keys.

"Don't you see? It is the ultimate validation of your theories," said Brozek. He could barely contain his glee. "Hungry people mindlessly follow orders. You feed them enough and right away they demand self-government."

The next day, September 13, Keys reversed his earlier decision and announced that the buddy system would be abandoned. For the first time since April, the men of Unit 115 could leave the stadium alone.

In some ways, the agitation of the men beneath the stadium mirrored the problems of the CPS as a whole. Many of the men in the CPS had been in for five years or more—like Lester Glick and Sam Legg. No end for the CPS men was in sight, even as soldiers were being mustered out of the service in droves. The lack of pay which at first had seemed to be a minor problem for a man taking a principled stand had grown into a major source of resentment. The lack of true "civilian direction" as promised by the Selective Service Act was also an ongoing source of aggravation.

The Historic Peace Churches for their part were growing tired of footing nearly the entire bill for a program of which they constituted barely half the membership. They mounted a campaign to shame the non–Historic Peace Churches into paying their share. In a widely distributed pamphlet, they made their claim directly, pointing out that the Historic Peace Churches had paid over a million dollars to fund the CPS service of men from churches not their own. The brochure then went into great embarrassing detail, actually showing the cost each non–Historic Peace Church had incurred, by way of supplying conscientious objectors in the CPS, compared to the amount of money contributed. The most indebted denomination, according to the brochure, was the Methodist Church, whose numerous conscientious objectors had cost the CPS $475,666 to maintain, while the Methodist Church had kicked in only $233,000. The Methodists were followed by the Jehovah's Witnesses and the Northern Baptists. The tone of the brochure was one of barely concealed frustration. As the war wound down, everyone was getting tired of the CPS.

This frustration reached its peak at Big Flats, New York, the camp that had been a prior home to several of the starvation guinea pigs. The CPS "union" in Big Flats that Max Kampelman had helped found had called for a general strike. Six men put down their shovels and axes and refused to work. They were joined by forty-seven COs who struck in sympathy at Camp 76 in Glendora, California. All were eventually arrested by the FBI. An organization called the Committee to End Slave Labor in America promoted their cause to anyone who would listen.

While many in Camp 115 in Minneapolis no doubt agreed that the CPS had flaws, they, in general, agreed with most of their peers that the CPS represented a great advance in the treatment of COs. The type of men who would volunteer for dangerous medical experiments were in general not the same type of radicals who agitated against the entire system. Many of the Minnesota men were personally aware of the treatment COs had received before the formation of the CPS. Harold Blickenstaff had grown up hearing stories of his father's prison sentence during World War I. The men also realized that in most other countries, their stance would have gotten them imprisoned or worse. By calling for the end to the buddy system, the COs in Minnesota were decidedly not calling for the dismantling of the CPS.

Football season began for the Golden Gophers of the University of Minnesota on September 22 with a game against Missouri. Minnesota's legendary coach, Bernie Bierman, had completed his alternative service as football coach to the navy cadets of the Iowa Preflight School. He returned to an adoring crowd of 34,246 fans eager to see him return Minnesota to glory, after having a 5-3-1 season under an interim coach in 1944. The men in the barracks beneath the stands heard the crowd cheer, an otherworldly roar that sounded like thunder, and the stomping of feet that sounded like torrential rain. They could also smell the hot dogs and the popcorn, smells that would have been unbearably tempting a few weeks earlier, before Keys had stepped up their rations. Even with their increased food, the guinea pigs were still tired. To those men who poked their heads out of the lab to watch the football game, the staged collisions of the giant men in helmets and pads struck them as an unforgivable waste of energy. Minnesota's Gophers won, 34–0. Some of the guinea pigs craned their necks to get a look at the cheerleaders on the sideline. Everywhere there were signs of recovery.

Intelligence was one of the attributes of the men most difficult to quantify, although that didn't stop Keys from trying. Keys tracked intelligence with both a battery of timed tests, and the CAVD test (completion, arithmetic, vocabulary, and directions), for which the men were allowed unlimited time; in starvation, they frequently took eight to ten hours to complete it. In neither test did starvation appear to significantly impact their abilities: "the measured intellective performance did not change importantly in either starvation or rehabilitation."

That result surprised no one more than the guinea pigs, who themselves felt that starvation had dulled their wits considerably. On the S24 complaint inventory, 28 percent of the men said their memories had worsened. Forty-one percent stated that they couldn't understand written materials as well as they had before the experiment. Keys attributed this self-evaluation to emotional distress. He couldn't argue with the independent, diverse intelligence tests that showed the men to be every bit as intelligent as when the study began.

Of course, intelligence was just one aspect of the mind that Keys wished to evaluate. Personality was another. He had asked Brozek to start assembling the psychological data for the men as they underwent their last round of tests for the study. He and Brozek were going over a stack of MMPI graphs when Brozek pointed excitedly to a particular file.

"Take a look at Subject 130," he said.

Keys thought for a moment. "Scholberg?"

"That's right. Look at this." Brozek pushed Scholberg's initial MMPI graph from the control phase across the desk. "Note the elevation here," said Brozek.

"On the psychotic end," said Keys. He remembered it well. Scholberg had been one of the subjects he was most worried about before the experiment began, both because of these elevated MMPI results and his frequently confessed fears for his own sanity.

"Now look at this," said Brozek. He was pushing a second graph for Scholberg across the desk. "This is from S24. Note the difference."

"The neurotic score has soared," said Keys. Again, not a big surprise—most of the men had seen their MMPI graphs veer towards the neurotic after six months of starvation.

"One more," said Brozek. "From the rehabilitation phase." This graph was strikingly different. All the scores were low, across the board.

"Everything's back to normal," said Keys.

"No!" said Brozek. "Not back to normal—better than normal. Much better than when the experiment began!"

"What does it mean?" said Keys.

"It means," said Brozek, "that for Henry Scholberg, this experiment has had quantifiable therapeutic value."

Keys continued to work feverishly on the interim report. His fear
that the recovery in Europe might be complete before the lab
could furnish any useable data spurred him on. With the
increased rations, the men were at last recovering, as graphs that
had for months sloped downwards began to rise. There was much
work to be done.

The original average weight in control was 152.7 pounds. The
average at the end of the starvation period was 115.6 pounds.
After twelve weeks in rehabilitation, the average weight had risen
to 129.2 pounds. The men had, in other words, regained only
36.7 percent of the weight they had lost in the experiment. Even
in the highest caloric group, the one that ended up receiving
2,400 calories a day more than they had in starvation, recovery
was not complete. The fortunate men in that group still weighed
on average about 10 percent less than when they first walked
through Gate 27 in November 1944.

Keys wanted his lab to study the functions of the human body
with the detachment and precision of an engineering laboratory
measuring the horsepower of a car engine. When he looked at the
big picture drawn by the thousands of tests, graphs, and X-rays
that they had created, Keys concluded that the human body was
supremely well equipped to deal with starvation. Eons of erratic
food supplies and natural disasters had built into the body an
array of mechanisms for conserving energy until the floodwaters
receded, the crops were restored, or the drought ended. In later
years Keys would say it was the most significant finding of the
study. The human body was very, very tough.

Keys wondered if the mind was as resilient. It certainly seemed
anecdotally that the mind of modern man, which viewed missing
a single meal as a tragedy, was less well equipped to deal with

long-term hunger. After a year, none of the men had been forced to quit because of their bodies giving out. Keys thought those tough young bodies probably had a lot more to give. It was the mind, in the end, that surrendered first. Keys thought of Legg lying in the hospital, those three circles of blood on his bandage.

But even Legg had pleaded to continue on. Keys thought about Kampelman trudging through the snow to class in the midst of starvation, and then fighting the good fight with the New York Bar's Committee on Character to boot. He thought about Scholberg on the verge of collapse, fearful for his own sanity, somehow finding the strength to finish what he started, and coming out the other side stronger than ever. Keys looked down at a pile of chest X-rays on his desk. He used them to measure the cardiac dimensions of each guinea pig. It was, he realized, an entirely inadequate method of evaluating a man's heart.

Keys published the interim report on October 15, 1945, just five days before the end of the experiment, but nearly five months after the end of the war in Europe. *Experimental Starvation in Man* at forty-eight pages was more than a pamphlet but something less than a comprehensive scientific report. In the first paragraph, Keys wrote, "There is at present in operation at the Laboratory of Physiological Hygiene an experimental study on human starvation and nutritional rehabilitation." He also wrote, "The subjects in this study are all conscientious objectors who were selected from volunteers in Civilian Public Service." He underlined the word *volunteers*. In the end, the report was largely descriptive, going into great detail about what starvation did to the human body. Because the rehabilitation phase was not complete, there was maddeningly little practical information Keys could convey to relief workers about treating the hungry. In all, the booklet devoted only ten lines to rehabilitation, mostly in the form of a promise for future information: "The results of the rehabilitation studies will be reported separately as the results are obtained and analyzed."

It was left to a member of the CPS to communicate the valuable insights they had to the relief workers of the world—Harold Guetzkow, the CPS psychologist who had been instrumental in first developing the idea of the starvation experiment with Keys. He wrote a seventy-page booklet entitled *Men and Hunger: A Psychological Manual for Relief Workers,* published by the Brethren Publishing House in Elgin, Illinois, in January 1946. The book was decidedly unscientific. Almost every page was illustrated with a cartoon. It was meant to provide specific, practical advice for relief workers, lessons gained during the experiment: *It is an unpardonable error for the (relief) worker to mention the dislike of any food. Above all, do not require people to stand in line for extended periods of time. Unnecessary exhibitions of strength and vitality on the part of others are a source of irritation. To see staff members take two stairs at a time was annoying to the men in our experiment.* In addition to being practical, Guetzkow's prose was occasionally artful. He compared an individual's rehabilitation to a *relived adolescence, a period of great awakening. His increased strength was wonderful, and often he underestimated his ability . . . Life experiences had a new freshness about them.*

Guetzkow's effort to put the hard-fought lessons of the experiment rapidly into a usable form was wholeheartedly endorsed by Keys, who wrote the foreword. There Keys explained again that it would be months before his voluminous data could be assembled into a complete scholarly text. In the meantime, he wrote, "it is our wish that practical application be made of the findings at both technical and non-technical levels. The present booklet is one means of bringing some of the facts to immediate use."

No one looked forward to the end of the experiment more than Lester Glick, the guinea pig who had been in the CPS the longest. Since June 23, 1941, Lester had been inside the Selective Service System, going from a forest service camp in Marietta, Ohio, to a mental hospital in Macedonia, Ohio, to another mental hospital in Ypsilanti, Michigan, to, finally, the starvation experiment. He had craved his mother's home cooking the entire time, but a year in Minneapolis had turned that homesickness into something of a desperate, unrequited love for food. Over the last few weeks of the experiment, Lester had meticulously compiled a list of twenty-nine different foods, and had somehow managed to scrape together the thirty dollars he estimated would buy them all. He'd make that purchase at the nearest grocery the second the experiment ended.

Like most of the volunteers, Lester's mood had soared with the increase in the diet after September 9, and the approaching end of their year together. He had worked hard, and he had made it. For the rest of his life, he would be able to say, I signed up for the toughest thing the CPS had to offer, and I made it to the finish line. A banquet was planned for October 20, the last day of the experiment, when the staff and the volunteers would eat one last meal together in Shevlin Hall to celebrate what they had accomplished.

On October 19, as Lester was cheerfully entertaining daydreams of buttered rolls and pickled beets, Dr. Taylor called him into his office. Glick was so cheerful that he thought nothing of it. He had once mentioned to the doctor that he might be interested in a career in medicine someday, and he thought that Taylor might want to offer some advice. Taylor shut the door as he entered.

"Lester, I've got some bad news." Glick noticed that there were X-rays on the doctor's desk. They had had regular chest X-rays since the beginning of the experiment. The doctor pointed to a white area on the image of Lester's left lung.

"This area is called the apex of your lung," the doctor said. "Do you see that spot?" He was pointing to a white anomaly on the film. Lester nodded, although it was hard for him to understand exactly what the doctor was talking about.

"That's a lesion," the doctor said. "Lester, I'm afraid you have tuberculosis."

Lester tried to take it all in. "Does that mean . . ." he said, "does that mean I can't be a doctor?" Taylor didn't respond. "Does this mean I can't go back to Sugar Creek?"

"Lester, you need to go to a sanitarium, and begin treatment— for a minimum of six months. This disease could kill you."

The next day the entire staff and the guinea pigs filed into Shevlin for their last, celebratory meal. Lester was determined to enjoy it. He had made it through the experiment after all, and starting tomorrow, he could eat whatever he wanted. Still, the unknown weighed heavily upon him, as he contemplated yet another delay before returning to Sugar Creek. The treatment would be expensive, no doubt, and he knew neither the CPS nor the Selective Service would be paying for any of it. His parents were farmers; he dreaded being a burden on them. Running underneath it all was the fear that the disease might result in something worse than six expensive months in a sanitarium.

Lost in such thoughts, it was a few moments before Lester Glick realized that he was sitting alone. Shevlin was crowded, with all the volunteers and the entire staff, but Glick had a table to himself. None of his comrades in the experiment could look him in the eye as they passed. He realized they had all heard the news about his tuberculosis and were afraid to sit next to him.

Lester looked down at his tray, his eyes stinging from the hurt. He wished he had skipped the meal altogether. He was a fool to think he could celebrate anything.

Suddenly, someone was standing across from him with a tray. "Lester?"

Lester looked up. It was Doctor Taylor. "May I join you?" he asked. Lester smiled.

The good doctor sat across from him, and soon others joined them at the table, which quickly became just as boisterous as any other in Shevlin Hall.

The experiment was over.

CHAPTER EIGHT

---◆◇◆---

THE HELSINKI DECLARATION

AS THE TEST SUBJECTS DRIFTED away from Minneapolis and toward normal meals, their interest in world events increased at roughly the same pace as their physical recovery. The timing was opportune, in a way, as the dark rumors of Nazi atrocities were suddenly thrust into broad daylight. The vivid testimony at the Nuremberg war crimes trials elicited conflicting responses from America's pacifists. Were the crimes of the Nazis so horrible that they justified a military response? Or were the Nazis the ultimate proof that militarism violates God's will for man? The test subjects of the starvation experiment, like the rest of the world, found that Nazism had twisted the morality of even those originally trained to heal and cure.

Twenty-three Nazis were tried at the Doctors' Trial at Nuremberg. Twenty were actually doctors, the other three bureaucrats in the vast Nazi medical establishment. They were accused by Brigadier General Telford Taylor, the American prosecutor, of "murders, tortures, and other atrocities committed in the name of medical science." Sixteen were found guilty, and seven of those were sentenced to hang on June 2, 1948. All were offered religious counsel in the days leading up to the hanging. Although the Nazi Party had scorned religion as a potentially dangerous distraction from one's duty to the state, only Karl Brandt declined the opportunity to speak to a clergyman.

Although he was known as Hitler's personal physician, the

industrious Brandt had found the time to participate in research projects throughout the war. Brandt was charged at Nuremberg with "special responsibility" for human experiments with pressure chambers, freezing, malaria, mustard gas, sulfanilamide, bone transplantation, sea water consumption, jaundice, sterilization with X-rays, and typhus. Brandt, like all of the doctors on trial, argued that his experiments on humans were part of a long and respected tradition in medicine, and were not in fact banned by any international law. If the defense at the 1946 Nuremberg trial of senior Nazi officers could be summed up as "I was just following orders," then the doctors' defense might be simplified as "researchers have always experimented on humans." The Nazis energetically gave examples of American medical experiments on prisoners, a population, they argued, that could not give the kind of absolute consent the American prosecutors insisted was necessary. The Nazis did not have to reach far back into history to make their point—a favorite example of the defense was the recent malaria experiment conducted on more than four hundred prisoners at Stateville Prison in Illinois.

The Stateville experiments took place from 1944 to 1945 over roughly the same time period as the starvation experiment. Photographs of the Stateville guinea pigs, in fact, appeared in the June 4, 1945, issue of *Life,* less than two months before the Wallace Kirkland photos of the starvation experiment were published for the same vast audience. The article is a good window on the public's perception of human experimentation at that time: "Men who have been imprisoned as enemies of society are now helping science fight another enemy of society." The article explained to readers why prisoners were such an ideal experimental group for the scientists: "Their subjects eat all the same food, sleep the same hours, and are never far away."

(One of the Stateville participants pictured in *Life* was Nathaniel Leopold, of the notorious murderous duo Leopold and Loeb. In his 1958 autobiography, *Life Plus 99 Years,* Leopold would say his work in the experiment was perhaps "just about as important" as actually fighting in the war. Indeed, Leopold devotes a whole chapter to his centrality in the experiments.)

The prosecution's expert witness on medical ethics, Dr. Andrew C. Ivy of the University of Illinois Medical School, said that no comparison could be made between the tortured Jews of Buchenwald and the prisoners of Stateville. He insisted that the prisoners in Illinois could be and were true volunteers. Moreover, Ivy outlined a series of general ethical standards for human experimentation that the Nazis had not met, starting with the quality of the science involved. The Stateville experiments had an important, clear, scientifically important goal: to find a cure for malaria. Many of the Nazi experiments were little more than thinly veiled sadism. Additionally, Ivy argued that experiments on humans must be based, to the maximum extent possible, on previous animal research. Finally, he said that experiments on humans should be conducted only by scientific experts.

Ivy cited a number of historical sources to prove that his standards were part of a long-accepted ethical tradition in medical research on humans. The Hippocratic oath, written between 470 and 360 B.C., was cited—it stated that the doctor's mandate was to work for the good of his patient. Dr. William Beaumont received credit for authoring the first American document dealing with the ethics of human experimentation in 1833, in which he stated that "the experiment is to be discontinued when it causes distress to the subject." Ironically, the first ethical code with the force of law behind it originated in Germany in 1900. This decree from the Prussian Minister of Religious, Educational, and Medical Affairs declared that experiments were forbidden if "the person concerned has not declared unequivocally that he consents to the intervention."

The American prosecution argued that many of the crimes of the Nazi doctors were in fact crimes even if there wasn't, strictly speaking, a formal international law that banned those specific acts at the time of their commission. The crimes of the Nazi doctors, the prosecution argued, were so horrible that any reasonable person would know they were wrong. They were, in effect, a violation of "natural" law.

After his conviction, Karl Brandt attempted to dodge the gallows by offering up his own living body to his American captors for medical experiments. No doubt the smug doctor thought he would prove something with this ironic self-sacrifice. He was surprised when his offer was declined.

As Keys had prophesied, World War II led to starvation on an epic scale. A flood of data and firsthand reports poured through Gate 27. From the Netherlands, from Greece, from the concentration camps, and from a score of other hungry locales came descriptions of every shade of hunger that can blight humanity. Keys regretted every delay in the publication of the complete starvation study, but he was determined to use it all. Keys wanted to do more than detail the twelve months of the experiment. He wanted to author the complete, seminal study of hunger, its history and every effect on the human body and mind.

While fulfilling that grand vision, Keys also had to get his Laboratory of Physiological Hygiene working on other projects. With the end of the war, the generous funding from the army was rapidly drying up. Finishing up the starvation study became an after-hours project, one that he worked on at night in his office and at home, as his family grew (third child Martha was born in 1949), and the starvation problem in Europe began to fade away.

In addition to incorporating all the latest reports from Europe, Keys wanted to fill the gaps in his study created by using an experimental set of exclusively young white males. Keys mentions the onset of amenorrhea among starving women as a parallel condition to the sexual impotence of starving men—in occupied Marseilles an estimated 70 percent of girls ceased having their menstrual periods. Similarly, the onset of menstruation was delayed among starving adolescent girls.

Keys also compiled data on anorexia nervosa, much of it showing that the disease is not an exclusively twentieth-century phenomenon. Keys obtained the 1895 autopsy of a sixteen-year-old girl who had died from anorexia nervosa weighing just 49 pounds. Keys noted that the Minnesota experiment actually more closely duplicated anorexia than it did wartime starvation, in that conditions other than food intake, such as cleanliness and accessibility of medical care, were "normal."

Keys also noted that in terms of starvation, women seemed more durable than men. The data came from across the globe and was remarkably consistent. In German-occupied Greece, males above the age of twenty died at much higher rates than females of the same age. In the Netherlands, during the famine of 1944–45, the mortality rate of females rose by 73 percent, while the rate for males rose 169 percent. In internment camps run by the Japanese, men made up 89.5 percent of all deaths deemed "natural" by the captors. Strikingly, one hundred percent of the suicides in one Japanese camp were men.

Keys listed several theories about the possible female advantages in starvation without endorsing any of them. Men require more food. Men continue to work longer after the onset of starvation. Women seek assistance sooner. Keys speculated that the "traditional woman's attitude of self-sacrifice and resignation" might be helpful. Not satisfied by any of those explanations, Keys stated, "Clearly, the whole question merits the closest scrutiny."

And even though the postwar hunger problem in Europe had largely passed him by, Keys did carefully document their findings and recommendations for relief workers in the final report. Up to a point, the results demonstrated that the pace of recovery was directly related to, and only to, the level of calories consumed. Neither the protein supplement nor the vitamin supplement had any appreciable effect on the rate or the degree of recovery. Keys was careful to point out that the experiment's basic rehabilitation diet, designed as it was to look like an actual European relief diet in the field, already contained a decent amount of protein, around 75 grams per day. In some other situation, Keys agreed, a small protein supplement might make a difference in the speed of recovery. However, Keys argued, "the relatively high cost of providing special protein feedings as compared with the cost of supplying additional calories far outweighs any possible advantage" that might be gained. Keys was unambiguous, aware that many people hoped or expected science to come up with a magical combination of proteins and vitamins that would hurry the rehabilitation process along. Such a potion didn't exist. He wrote, "We do not wish to qualify our conclusion that the calorie intake is the single nutritional element of highest importance in rehabilitation feeding of persons starved on a European type of famine diet."

The reports Keys included from the concentration camps were among the most compelling sections of the study, a chilling contrast to the sterile data from the lab. "The situation," Keys wrote, "was worse than had been believed possible even from the most somber predictions, and the conditions for trying out the procedures [for rehabilitation] were far from satisfactory. Belsen was entered on April 17, 1945, and some 50,000 inmates, together with 8,000 to 10,000 unburied dead, were found in the most incredible state of emaciation. In the first days there were about 300 deaths a day."

Relief workers had prepared to nourish victims through intravenous and oral tube feeding on a massive scale, in the belief that among the severely starved, the digestive tract would be too deteriorated to sustain normal eating and digestion. Not so, said Keys. "The vast majority of the famine victims could take nourishment by mouth without any special difficulty." Relief workers found this to be true even for the severely emaciated. There were sobering nonmedical reasons for simple oral feeding as well:

many camp survivors were understandably reluctant to participate in anything that looked remotely like a science experiment.
"The Belsen patients considered stomach tubes a new form of tor-
ture," wrote Keys. Normal feeding was the superior method in
almost all cases. To relief workers, freed from the burden of
transporting and operating elaborate tube and intravenous feeding apparatus, Keys wrote that the information should be "a
cause for rejoicing."

Finally, in 1950, it was done. Published by the University of
Minnesota Press, *The Biology of Human Starvation* was a massive, two volume, 1,385-page work that was immediately hailed
as the seminal work on the subject of starvation. The scale of the
book reflected Keys' outsized ambition. The first chapter, written
in part by Max Kampelman, was devoted to the history of starvation, a history that stretched back as far as there were records of
man's struggles on earth. A seven-year famine in Egypt starting in
1708 B.C. was the oldest referred to. Everything about the study
was monumental. It contained four forewords, two indices, and
565 data tables: Table 565 listed the exact contents of the Cooperative for American Remittances to Europe (CARE) package, all
40,000 calories. The bibliography went on for eighty-six single-
spaced pages, citing more than 2,800 sources, ranging from J.
Penkethman's 1748 work, *A True Relation or Collection of the
most Remarkable Dearths and Famines which have happened
within this Realme since the Coming in of William the Conquerer,*
to the thirty-seven-page operating manual for the Maico
audiometer. The guinea pigs were offered discounted copies of the
study; almost all took advantage of the offer.

Only the timing of the publication kept it from being an
unqualified triumph. Sir Jack Drummond wrote in his foreword,
"My admiration was tinted with only one regret, that the investi-
gation had not begun three years earlier." Keys agreed in his own
foreword, "We regret, of course, that this work was not published when the hunger of the world was more acute than now."

In recognizing that the immediate problems of starvation had been ameliorated, Keys had aimed for a much higher target. He wanted the study to be the comprehensive reference on one of mankind's most fundamental problems. If it couldn't be done in time to use in the refugee camps that sprang up immediately after the war, Keys wanted to publish a book that would be used by doctors and scientists for decades to come. Only time would tell if he had been successful.

The judges at Nuremberg rejected the main defense of the Nazi doctors that there had been no international standard prohibiting them from conducting their experiments on humans. The tribunal then sought to eliminate that argument from any future trials by creating a formal code. Drawing on both modern conceptions and ancient ethical precedents, and relying heavily on the input of Dr. Ivy, they created the landmark Nuremberg Code. It was the first assertion by any body of an international standard governing medical experimentation on humans. At the same time it was an assertion by society that doctors could no longer be trusted to police themselves.

The distrust was short-lived, if it ever existed at all in the United States. Doctors proclaimed that they were bound by the tight cords of their own personal and professional ethics, making the Nuremberg Code unnecessary. Americans wanted to believe them. In addition, many researchers found the Nuremberg Code too burdensome, especially the first clause that mandated absolute consent from test subjects, the type of consent that would preclude the use of prisoners, the insane, children, or the incompetent. Perhaps most fundamentally, American doctors believed that the Nuremberg Code was written for deranged Nazi doctors, not them. American physicians were the scientific descendants of Walter Reed and Jonas Salk, not of Mengele and Karl Brandt. So the Nuremberg Code was largely ignored as research on humans continued on in the United States just as it always had, regulated almost completely by the personal ethics of the physicians in charge.

Incredibly, this was true even for one of the framers of the Nuremberg Code, Dr. Andrew Ivy, the Nuremberg prosecution's expert witness on medical ethics. In the years after the war, Ivy became enamored of a worthless experimental cancer drug derived from horse blood and known as "Krebiozen." Despite numerous scientific reports showing that it had no curative value, Ivy enthusiastically treated hundreds of cancer patients with the drug. Ridiculed as a quack, he was forced to resign as vice president of the University of Illinois in 1953, but he continued to experiment with Krebiozen on cancer patients until his death in 1976.

In the years after the Doctors' Trial, after the tenets of informed consent and ethical experimentation had supposedly been written in stone, doctors in rural Alabama continued to allow a cadre of unknowing African-American men to suffer syphilis untreated so they could track the disease's progress all the way through autopsy. The study was sponsored by the United States Public Health Service—and was not a secret. The progress of the experiment had been reported often in medical journals and discussed at conferences ever since its inception in 1932. Most of the doctors involved would maintain until the very end that they had done nothing wrong. The experiment would end in 1972 only after a torrent of bad press exposed the details to a horrified public.

In the years after Nuremberg prohibited it, experimentally exposing unknowing human beings to radiation grew into a veritable industry in the United States. The goal of these federally sponsored Cold War experiments was usually to determine the effects of various kinds of radiation on the body in anticipation of an all-out nuclear war with the Soviet Union. The scale of the experimentation boggles the mind: an investigative panel formed in the 1990s found that over four thousand separate experiments had been conducted, many of which flaunted the ethical standards established at Nuremberg. Between the late 1940s and 1961, mentally retarded children institutionalized at the Fernald State School in Massachusetts were exposed to radiation, having been enticed into the experiment with extra milk and membership in a "science club." Between 1960 and 1972, cancer patients at the University of Cincinnati were unnecessarily exposed to total-body irradiation, after being told it was a treatment for their illness. In fact, they were participating in a risky Department of Defense study. Between 1945 and 1965, from 500,000 to 2.3 million school children throughout the country took part in nasal radium experiments. Investigators later estimated that these children would go through life with a 62 percent increased chance of developing deadly tumors in the central nervous system.

Other examples of the inadequacy or the irrelevancy of the Nuremberg Code are distressingly easy to find. Beginning in 1956, retarded children at the Willowbrook State School for the Retarded on Staten Island, New York, were injected with hepatitis. Without completely disclosing the details of the study, scientists offered expedited admission to the school for cooperative parents who would give their consent. In 1986, Saul Krugman, the lead researcher, still maintained that the study was ethical. In 1963, researchers at the Brooklyn Jewish Chronic Disease Hospital injected impoverished elderly patients with live cancer cells without their consent. In 1974, the Pharmaceutical Manufacturers Association of America estimated that about 70 percent of approved drugs had at some point been tested on prisoners.

With each disclosure, the public became less trusting of science and scientists. The Atomic Age that had seemed so hopeful and bright turned ominous and dark. While the doctors maintained that their research was both necessary and ethical, the public couldn't help but notice that the test subjects almost always seemed to be among society's most vulnerable, like poor southern blacks, retarded children, the elderly, and the incarcerated. In response, and to fend off anything beyond self-regulation, the World Medical Association created a new set of standards for experimentation on humans at its eighteenth World Medical Assembly in Helsinki, Finland, in June 1964.

The Helsinki Declaration was at the same time less rigorous but more effective than the Nuremberg Code. Less rigorous because it watered down the absolute nature of the "voluntary consent" clause that was the first principle of the Nuremberg Code, the restriction seen as the most onerous by researchers. Unlike Nuremberg, the Helsinki Declaration makes room for incapacitated and incompetent subjects, requiring only that consent be procured from legal guardians. The Helsinki Declaration also divided research into two broad classifications: nontherapeutic and therapeutic. Therapeutic research is research undertaken while trying to treat a sick person. The declaration paints this kind of experimentation in positive, almost heroic terms: "In the treatment of the sick person the doctor must be free to use a new therapeutic measure if in his judgment it offers hope of saving life, re-establishing health, or alleviating suffering."

The Helsinki Declaration is more effective than the Nuremberg Code most of all because it has the endorsement of the global medical community. While the Nuremberg Code was a legal document largely seen as a set of guidelines for barbarian Nazi doctors, the Helsinki Declaration was created by the physicians of the world. The Helsinki Declaration is also more effective because modern society demands limits on experimentation. People believe more now than they did in the late 1940s that research on humans must be regulated by something other than the individual doctor's conscience.

Could the Minnesota Starvation Experiment be conducted today? Most of the people alive today who were connected with the experiment reflexively say no, that today, the Helsinki Declaration would not allow it. In fact, the Helsinki Declaration is much more ambiguous than that. The Helsinki Declaration does allow nontherapeutic research, given that consent is obtained and risks explained, all of which Ancel Keys did on his own. Some might make the case that the risks were unknown, but of course this is always true to some extent; that is why scientists conduct experiments. Some might also argue about the quality of the consent given by the CPS men. They were, after all, compelled by the Selective Service System to do something. There were many alternatives, however, and even now, knowing all that they know, the surviving test subjects almost all say they would volunteer to do it again. Dr. David Smith, a psychologist at the University of Notre Dame, says the experiment would never be allowed by modern ethical guidelines. Dr. Henry Keys, son of Ancel and a cancer researcher, says it could be.

But all agree that the argument is completely academic. The experiment could never be conducted today because no scientist could ever gather together thirty-six men willing to live under a football stadium for a year without pay in order to lose a quarter of their body weight. Ethical guidelines are organic, flexible things that adjust with the times and the needs of society. The circumstances that made the starvation experiment possible will never happen again.

And that is what has made the study so valuable. Keys wanted to conduct the experiment because nothing like it had ever been done before. He could not have known that it would never be done again. The study remains the definitive work on the subject, and is constantly referenced in scientific works on nutrition and hunger. For researchers looking for hard, controlled, scientific data on the effects of starvation on the human body and mind, there is nowhere else to turn. Those 1,385 pages are the lasting monument to the starvation experiment.

While called upon by doctors of many different disciplines, *The Biology of Human Starvation* is especially useful to researchers of anorexia nervosa. As Keys himself said in the study, the Minnesota experiment more closely duplicated the conditions of anorexics than it did concentration camp prisoners. The study is invaluable for those treating anorexics because it helps separate the symptoms that are a result of anorexia from those that are just byproducts of hunger. The hunger must be treated first. As one anorexia researcher wrote after citing the characteristics of starvation noted by Keys: "Trying to make meaningful psychological changes with an anorexic patient in this starved state is analogous to trying to address underlying issues with an alcoholic patient who is intoxicated."

Just as Keys' life bridged the worlds between high science and popular culture, so too do those who cite the starvation experiment. Dr. Arthur Agatston refers to Keys' work in the *South Beach Diet*—although he repeatedly misspells Keys' name as "Ansel." Historians, too, have often attempted to explain the strange behavior of the starving throughout history with the insights gained in Minnesota. In his book *In the Heart of the Sea,* historian Nathaniel Philbrick quotes a sea captain who thought the cannibalism of his shipwrecked crew had caused their savage behavior: "their eyes staring and looking wild, their countenances fierce and barbarous." In fact, Philbrick points out, the coarse behavior of the men was a normal response to starvation, as shown in the Minnesota Starvation Experiment. Gavan Daws in *Prisoners of the Japanese* compares the hunger of the CPS men in Minnesota to the privations suffered by Allied prisoners in the Pacific Theater. In *The Mapmaker's Wife,* Robert Whitaker refers to the experiment when explaining exactly how starvation consumed the bodies of his protagonists in the Amazon. Historians, like scientists, have had only one comprehensive source of information on the subject of starvation.

CHAPTER NINE

THE COVER OF *TIME*

As he studied the final drafts of *The Biology of Human Starvation,* Keys noticed something curious in the mortality data pouring in from Europe. In the Netherlands, where the food deprivation had been among the worst in Europe during the war, heart attack rates were actually dropping. At this same time, heart disease was reaching almost epidemic proportions among American men. Heart disease had, in fact, been the leading cause of death in the United States since 1921. Keys himself noticed while scanning the Minneapolis obituary pages that heart disease seemed to be stalking all the high-ranking businessmen of the Twin Cities. Keys theorized that the intake of fatty foods was somehow related to the high incidence of heart disease. He also knew that recent research had shown a link between fat consumption and levels of cholesterol in the blood. Keys' research would unite those theories, make him famous, and make cholesterol a household word.

Years later, Keys would describe cholesterol as "an important and remarkable substance quite apart from its unfortunate tendency to be deposited in the walls of arteries." Keys was concerned with total cholesterol—its separation into "good" and "bad" varieties was years away. Chemically, cholesterol is described by the formula $C_{27}H_{46}OH$. While it is waxy looking, it is not a fat—cholesterol is a complex alcohol, a member of a group of compounds known as sterols. The word *cholesterol* is derived from the Greek words for "solid bile," which speaks to the fact that cholesterol is manufactured by the body in the liver. The body manufactures cholesterol because it is an important component of brain cells and nerve cells. It is also used by the body to make nonsoluble fats soluble, so that they can be carried about the body in the bloodstream. Even before his study began, Keys theorized that this "remarkable substance," overproduced by the body because of a fatty diet, might be playing a role in the plague of heart attacks that seemed to be afflicting the world's rich and well-fed.

Keys began his research in 1946 by persuading 286 Minneapolis executives to participate in a long-term research project that would involve periodic exhaustive exams at the lab for the rest of their lives. Always adept at managing publicity, Keys invited Edward John Thye, the state's Republican governor, to take part, as well as beloved Minnesota football coach Bernie Bierman. Both accepted. The study would attempt to measure over the years the effects of several factors on mortality, with special attention focused on diet, cholesterol, and heart disease.

As Keys explored the epidemiology of chronic heart disease, not all his research subjects were well-fed Minneapolis businessmen. Keys wanted a more controlled group, one in which he could do more than passively measure and record data. He wanted to actively manipulate the diet, control variables, and measure changes—a scenario he was accustomed to. The availability of CPS guinea pigs had ended with the war, so Keys turned to a friend, Dr. Ralph Rosen, at Hastings State Hospital. Keys was allowed to plan the diets for thirty patients divided into two groups. Hastings State was a hospital for the insane.

"Our dietary experiments could do no harm," wrote Keys years later. "Indeed, we were to see the men respond favorably to our attention to them; they became slightly less apathetic." The two diets provided to the group were exactly the same except for fat content. Caloric equality was maintained in the low fat diet by exchanging starches for fat. Keys proved convincingly with his mentally ill test subjects that meat fat raised the cholesterol level in the blood. Keys was off and running.

Because of the sheer scale of the problem, Keys wanted to look at coronary heart disease from an epidemiological point of view; that is, to study relatively isolated populations in an attempt to identify risk factors in each. With data from his Minnesota businessmen already being accumulated, Keys turned his eyes toward a country known for having one of the highest incidences of heart disease—Finland—and one with one of the lowest—Japan. Anecdotal evidence from those countries certainly seemed to support Keys' theories. The Japanese lived on a diet of fish and rice, virtually devoid of saturated fats. Finns in lumber camps, Keys witnessed with amazement, would often slather butter onto a thick slice of cheese for lunch.

Keys' plan for Finland and Japan mirrored his study of Minneapolis executives: men aged forty to fifty-nine would be given rigidly standardized physical exams at five-year intervals. As Keys traveled the world collecting data and proselytizing about the dangers of a fatty diet, he gained allies in the international medical community. By 1956, four other nations had joined in the study: Greece, Yugoslavia, Italy, and the Netherlands. The project would become known as the Seven Countries Study.

Keys' epidemiological approach to the study of heart disease was encouraged by another celebrity scientist: President Eisenhower's personal physician, Paul Dudley White. The fatherly doctor had nursed the president back to health after his 1955 heart attack, an achievement for which he won the lasting affection of the American people. He was also an esteemed cardiologist, a founder of the American Heart Association in 1924, and elected president of the same group in 1941. Like Keys, he was an early prophet of the links between lifestyle and heart disease. A staunch advocate of exercise, he once walked from National Airport to the White House for an appointment with the president. In Keys,

White saw a kindred spirit. His endorsement of Keys' work opened many doors at home and abroad.

The study would take Keys and his family on an international odyssey, making him friends in communities around the world. Keys preferred to work in rural villages, where populations were relatively isolated, stable, and could be examined in almost their entirety. The nature of his work led to an unending stream of interesting medical revelations. In Nicotera, Italy, in 1957, Keys examined the local death records and found six men whose cause of death was *gelosia*—the Italian word for "jealousy." He found out later that they had all been shot. In a mountain village in Crete, Keys saw old farmers working in the field who drank only a glass of olive oil for breakfast; he later verified that one of them was 106 years old. In all, Keys accumulated data on over 12,000 men around the world. Keys' two oldest children, Carrie and Henry, were often ensconced in boarding school, but Margaret and baby Martha accompanied him on his travels, which became a grand family adventure.

Of the seven countries studied, Finland, home of the buttered cheese, had the highest incidence of heart attack deaths: 992 out of 10,000 deaths. Crete in Greece, where people lived on fresh vegetables and olive oil, had the lowest incidence: just 9 out of 10,000. Interestingly, both countries consumed roughly equal amounts of fat: about 40 percent of their total caloric intake. The difference was that in Finland, those fat calories were largely of the saturated variety, the kind of fat associated with meat and dairy.

Some of the results were surprising. Even in the fifties, smoking was a widely recognized risk factor in heart disease. Keys found that in comparison to cholesterol, the effect of smoking was minor. His test groups in Japan and Crete had among the highest percentage of people smoking a pack a day or more—43 percent in Japan, 30 percent in Crete. But these locales had among the lowest heart attack rates—which directly correlated with their extremely low cholesterol levels. It appeared to Keys that elevated cholesterol had to be present first, before smoking could increase risk.

Another counterintuitive result of the study was that high cholesterol foods in the diet were not a major contributing factor to cholesterol in the blood. The amount of saturated fat in the diet, which stimulated the liver to produce its own cholesterol, was in fact the major predictor of blood cholesterol level. Keys was even able to develop a formula which accurately predicted cholesterol level in the blood based on diet. The "Keys Formula" is still in wide use today.

To Keys, the connection between high cholesterol and high levels of coronary heart disease was clear. To demonstrate this relationship, Keys constructed a dramatic graph that plotted deaths from heart disease against percentage of fat calories consumed for several different countries in the study. The result was an almost perfectly straight line on a semi-logarithmic graph with Japan at the very bottom of the curve and the United States perched at the very top. The graph showed with mathematical certainty that a diet high in fat led directly to a population with more heart attacks. One medical historian would call it "one of the most widely published and republished graphs in the literature relating to coronary heart disease, its etiology, prevention, and treatment." Later researchers would criticize Keys for omitting data he had in hand from countries that didn't conform to his dramatic curve, but Keys felt no need to apologize. Keys was confident in his thesis, and the graph was a powerful representation of his theory to all who saw it. Let lesser scientists quibble about graphing additional dots—he was trying to save America. Keys had no qualms about using the sheer scale of his study as a bludgeon against those who questioned his theories. "I've got five thousand cases," he was known to say to critics. "How many do you have?"

To Keys, the entire population of the United States, made fat by habit and prosperity, was sick. A person on the low end of the spectrum for blood cholesterol in the United States would have very high cholesterol in Japan. To make a change, Keys knew, he was going to have to reach out beyond the medical journals and scientific conferences. He needed to convince all of America to change the way it looked at food and nutrition. The U.S. population was his patient, and he had a duty to act. "If some countries can do without heart attacks," he asked, "why can't we?"

Keys got an idea how he might reach a broader audience during his frequent trips to southern Italy for the Seven Countries Study. Keys had grown fond of the food of southern Italy as a young man in California's Bay Area, where many Italian immigrants had settled—he was a lifelong lover of pasta. The abundance of fresh vegetables in southern Italy was also reminiscent of the beloved cuisine of his youth.

What Keys had learned as a scientist was that the southern Italian diet he enjoyed so much was also extremely healthy. The people of southern Italy tended to have very low cholesterol, and coronary heart disease was almost unknown. While the data for the Seven Countries Study would be accumulated for decades, Keys thought he had enough information about diet and heart disease to communicate it to the public immediately. He would do so in the form of a cookbook cowritten with wife Margaret. The book would explain to lay people the scientific basis for a Mediterranean-style diet, and provide American consumers with practical and palatable recipes. Keys wrote the scientific portions of the book, while Margaret tried out recipes on their friends and neighbors. Paul Dudley White wrote the foreword: "It is a happy blending of the scientific aspects of nutrition, the hazards of over-nutrition, and the pleasures of the table." The resulting book, *Eat Well and Stay Well,* was a sensation.

Published by Doubleday & Company in 1959, the book would eventually be translated into five languages and sell well over one hundred thousand copies. It was far from a typical cookbook.

The first recipe didn't appear until page 216: Connecticut cottage cheese. Everything before was devoted to explaining in straightforward terms the links between cholesterol—"a greasy or waxy substance, essentially tasteless and odorless"—and coronary heart disease—"the condition produced by interference with the blood flow in the arteries that supply the heart muscle itself." The book makes one fleeting reference to the starvation experiment, in a chapter on losing weight: "This is an extreme case of adaptation by men who were not fat to begin with but who lost a fourth of their original body weight." He also took a preemptive shot at his peers who might look down their noses at writing a cookbook: "Some of these believe practically nothing is provable and that scientific research is fun so long as you do not seriously expect it to produce useful results."

The book introduced Middle America to paella, gnocchi, and gazpacho. While the book had a heavy emphasis on Mediterranean cuisine, Keys also encouraged his fellow Americans to try the food of the Chinese, "who take second place to none in cookery." The Chinese restaurant owners of America repaid the endorsement by exhibiting window streamers and counter cards advertising the book.

The royalties from the book allowed Keys and Margaret to build Minnelea, a magnificent villa on the Mediterranean in the village of Pioppi, one hundred miles south of Naples. With a terrace on the sea, a tiled roof, and a citrus garden, it was worlds away from the gray house on Shattuck Avenue in Berkeley where Keys grew up. At first, it was just Keys' sun-drenched retreat from the long Minneapolis winter, but with each passing year he and Margaret spent more time on the Mediterranean, and less time in frigid Minnesota.

With Keys' wartime work and the publication of a bestselling cookbook, he very much fit the mold of the great American hero-scientist, an archetype created by America's postwar, post–Manhattan Project faith in science and scientists. Men such as Albert

Einstein and Jonas Salk were the archetypes. Like those two men, Keys would receive on January 13, 1961, exactly one week before President John F. Kennedy's inauguration, the mark of modern American fame. He was pictured on the cover of *Time* magazine. He was the only University of Minnesota faculty member, before or since, to ever be so honored.

The *Time* article was entitled "The Fat of the Land," and it mostly dwelt on Keys' two main themes since the war: (1) Americans eat too much, and (2) Americans eat too much fat. The magazine also described Keys in the style of a celebrity profile, so that readers might learn about the man as well as his theories. His boyhood work in the guano cave was explained, as was Keys' remarkable rise through the academic ranks. The article related Keys' height (5 feet 7 inches), his normal breakfast (half a grapefruit), and how to make a negroni, his favorite cocktail: 1/4 gin, 1/4 Campari bitters, 1/4 sweet or dry vermouth, and 1/4 soda water, over ice in an old-fashioned glass. Readers learned that Keys ate slowly, but drove fast, in a two-toned Karmann-Ghia. The article mentioned the K ration, the Seven Countries Study, and the cookbook. It made no mention of the starvation experiment.

Not everyone was happy with Keys' theories about cholesterol, especially as they were jumping from the academic journals into America's popular press. This unhappy group included some of Keys' old patrons. The National Dairy Council, which had provided part of the funding for the starvation experiment, became one of the main naysayers of Keys' work linking high fat diets to high cholesterol in the blood and heart disease. Keys brushed off their criticism and continued to charge headlong into the battle.

While Keys was unwilling to acknowledge his increasing years in his workload or his travel schedule, he was interested in the physiological effects of aging. In 1962, Keys organized a high-altitude study on California's White Mountain, in the Inyo-White

Mountains near the Nevada border. It was an expedition of graying scientists: Keys was the youngest at 58, the oldest was 72. The mountains were home to the White Mountain Research Station, a facility run by the University of California. The main structure there was named the Barcroft Facility, after Keys' onetime mentor at Cambridge. Keys' study at the summit of White Mountain, at 14,246 feet, took place twenty-six years after he hustled his way to the top of the frozen Chilean Andes. One unpublished result of the study did seem to show that some psychological mellowing takes place with aging—Keys did not deck any of his fellow scientists on the 1962 expedition.

The Keyses published another bestselling cookbook in 1967, and on this one Margaret took top billing: *The Benevolent Bean,* again published by Doubleday. This book would be lighter on the medical science and heavier on recipes, and sell well again, earning the Keyses more fame and more royalties. Ancel Keys was America's nutritionist laureate. He was passionate, and much to the delight of the press, he was eminently quotable. "Americans have Sunday dinner every day," he grumbled. Heart disease was caused, he said, "by the North American habit of turning the stomach into the garbage disposal unit for a long list of harmful foods." Although fellow scientists occasionally groused among themselves about his simplifications, Americans appreciated Keys' explanations of these complex, worrisome issues. It was never grandstanding to Keys. He regarded it as his moral duty to put his findings into the public forum, beyond the stuffy club of professional journals where his research would have little effect on his "patient"—the entire population of the United States.

Keys retired from the University of Minnesota in 1972. He was succeeded as head of the Laboratory of Physiological Hygiene by friend and protégé Henry Blackburn. At Keys' retirement dinner, Blackburn would give about as good a description of Keys as anyone who knew him: "Ancel Keys has a quick and brilliant mind, and great perseverance. He can also be frank to the point of blunt trauma, and critical to the point of a razor slash." While Keys was retired, his world travel continued unabated as he continued his quest for data and preached the gospel of low cholesterol.

A torrent of data from the Seven Countries Study poured in. In all, 12,763 men between the ages of forty and fifty-nine were given baseline examinations between 1958 and 1964. Repeat medical exams were given at five and ten years after baseline. Twenty-five years after the baseline exam, a "mortality follow up" was conducted. In all, 5,973 of the middle-aged men had died within twenty-five years of their baseline exam. Of those, about 1,500 had died of coronary heart disease. In large part, the statistics bore out the theory Keys had spelled out decades before—that a fatty diet led to high cholesterol, which lead to heart disease. It was a tribute to Keys' proselytizing that by the time the final results were known after twenty-five years, those conclusions were already largely accepted as fact.

Memorial Stadium was not showing its age as well as Keys in the 1970s. The laboratory was moved from the stadium to the comparatively sterile Health Sciences Unit A on the Twin Cities campus. In 1981, the university's board of regents voted against spending the $10 million necessary to bring the stadium up to modern code, and moved the Golden Gophers football games to the newly constructed and equally sterile Hubert H. Humphrey Metrodome downtown, starting with the 1982 season. There were some spirited fights to preserve the old stadium, but the football team's move was the death knell. The class of 1942 carted the memorial arch and sculpture away for storage. The rest of the stadium was demolished in 1992. Dr. Keys and his children Henry and Carrie watched the wrecking balls from within sight of Gate 27. Keys was twenty years older than the stadium they were demolishing.

Ancel Keys' long and notable career guaranteed a generation of scientific descendants, two of them in the most literal sense. For those growing up in the Keys household, a career in the medical sciences was practically assumed. Ancel used to hold up chicken bones at the dinner table and ask the children to name the bone and its human counterpart. Henry Keys grew up observing both his father, the hard-nosed scientist, and his maternal grandfather, the quintessential family doctor from Duluth, Minnesota. Henry as a boy once asked his father why he chose research over being a medical doctor. Ancel replied, "I could never be a bedside hand-shaker." Henry was undeterred and became a physician, as well as a cancer researcher. Daughter Carrie became a clinical psychologist, a career path to which Ancel also offered a characteristically gruff critique: "How do you know when you've done any good? A clinical psychologist can't measure anything." Both son and daughter are widely respected in their fields.

Keys outlived his youngest child. Young Martha, who as a small girl braved her parents' scientific odyssey across Europe, was shot through the heart by thieves while on a family vacation in Jamaica in 1991. She was 42; Ancel was 87. At her funeral, Keys found himself too crushed to stand during the sermon. His old eyes, he wrote later, had run out of tears.

Reluctantly, Keys began to make concessions to age. He and Margaret gave up their beloved villa in Italy in 2001; the travel had become too difficult. They moved into an assisted-living facility in Minneapolis. The apartment was crowded with memories—his elaborate Cambridge cap and gown hung in the closet. The small table he had haggled for on the docks of Hong Kong over seventy years earlier sat in a corner of the kitchen. And everywhere there were books—books he had written, books written by his students, books written about his work. As his eyesight faded, Margaret would read to him, but the loss of reading was a terrible blow. "My room is filled with books I cannot read," he wrote on an oversized word processor designed for those with poor vision. "The words are only spots that spoil the page."

Journalists would stop by occasionally, wanting to meet the namesake of the K ration. They always wanted him to link his own longevity to his theories on nutrition, but he refused to. An uncompromising scientist to the end, Keys insisted that you couldn't draw that kind of inference from his life, a single case. You needed mathematical analysis and a large sample size, perhaps even five thousand cases, before you could correlate his personal diet to his one hundred years on earth.

On September 12, 2004, an esteemed international group of experts on nutrition gathered at the Minneapolis Hilton for the First International Ancel Keys Symposium on Nutrition and Health. The subject of the symposium was the international obesity epidemic. If anyone noticed the irony of the obesity symposium being named for the world's foremost expert on starvation, it was not mentioned. Ancel Keys, the guest of honor, was one hundred years old.

All the scientific presentations were scheduled for Day 2. September 12, a Sunday, was an all-day celebration of the long career of Dr. Keys. Such unabashed sentimentality had to be smuggled into a serious academic symposium, otherwise Keys would probably never have allowed it. The day featured talks by family, friends, and old colleagues. They spoke with the conviction of old friends eager to show the "other" side of their gruff guest of honor.

Sunday ended with Dixieland jazz performed by Henry Blackburn's combo—Keys' successor at the Laboratory of Physiological Hygiene was also a talented clarinetist. On Monday, it was on to the serious business of obesity, a full day of lectures with names like "The Development of Obesity: Macronutrients vs. Calories" and "Interactions between Adipose Tissue and Energy Metabolism." As always, it was hard to gauge Keys' reaction, but all in all, he seemed more comfortable with the science than with the heartfelt tributes of a day earlier.

————————

Ancel Keys died ten weeks later.

CHAPTER TEN

---◇---

UNRESTRICTED REHABILITATION

NOT ALL THE GUINEA PIGS were in headlong rush to leave the laboratory at the conclusion of the experiment. Dr. Keys managed to get twelve volunteers to stay at the lab for another eight weeks after R12, a group that included Max Kampelman. Keys called the phase "Unrestricted Rehabilitation," meaning that although their diets were unsupervised, science needed to occasionally take a look at them to analyze the lasting effects of the experiment. In that sense, it was a phase most of the men would live in for the rest of their lives.

During that first unrestricted week, R13, twelve very hungry young men were unloosed on the Twin Cities. They each consumed on average 5,219 calories per day. Most commented that even when they were stuffed to the point that they couldn't eat any more, they still felt hungry. Psychological aftereffects were also noted. There was a seldom-verbalized irrational fear among them that food might be again taken away. Periodic uncontrolled gorging was common. The doctors noted with awe that Richard Mundy, on one Saturday in November, managed to consume 11,500 calories. The unrestricted phase ended after eight weeks, on December 20, 1945. There would be two more follow-up testing periods, one in March 1946 (R33) and one in August 1946 (R55).

There would also be unofficial follow-ups. At a 1991 guinea pig reunion hosted by Charles Smith in St. Petersburg, Florida,

Lester Glick handed out a questionnaire asking the sixteen guinea pigs in attendance to evaluate their experience in Minnesota some fifty years earlier. Glick had in the intervening decades received a doctorate in social work, and was a dean at Goshen College, a Mennonite College in Indiana. He was well versed in the objective application of research and statistics. Still, it was possible to see the painful imprint of the experiment in Glick's questions to his peers. More than 80 percent agreed with Glick's statement: "The experiment increased my capacity to cope with adversity." Despite this, more than 60 percent said they would encourage their own sons to participate in a similar experiment. Many of the men said that the experiment was the most important experience of their lives. Glick's sense of humor was also on display in the survey—he asked if a love of macaroni and cheese was a long-term effect of the experiment. Many agreed that it was.

In 1998, Dr. Scott Crow and a colleague at the University of Minnesota decided to conduct perhaps the last scientific survey of the starvation guinea pigs. It was understood that not too many opportunities to work with these men remained. The test subjects' average age in 1944 had been 25, making that average volunteer 79 in 1998. Dr. Crow was able to locate 19 of the original 36 guinea pigs. Eleven were known dead; 6 could not be found.

Dr. Crow came to the starvation study as an expert in eating disorders. His questioning of the starvation subjects reflected this interest. Crow was fascinated to find that just like anorexics, the men in the experiment had at times greatly distorted body images. During the starvation phase, many of the men thought that people not in the experiment looked fat, especially the staff they saw every day. They also seemed unaware of their own skeletal appearance. During rehabilitation, some of the men complained that they "felt fat." Crow found that most of the men had exceeded their control period weight significantly in the years after the experiment, by an average of 27 pounds. Gradually, though, over a period of years, most men drifted back to their original weight. In Crow's study, only three of the men said they never again got back down to their original control weight.

What impressed Crow most in his look at these men, what seemed to him to be their salient abnormal feature in relation to the general population, was their high level of achievement. Crow speculated that the rigorous original screening for the experiment had successfully managed to select an extraordinary group, a group perhaps more resistant to pain and more willing to sacrifice than the population at large. There was the additional fact that the men had been screened initially for an ability to get along well with others, a characteristic that may also have well predicted later success. The impressive resumes of the men were impossible to deny, even if "success" over the course of a long life can be a tricky thing for a scientist to attempt to quantify. When Crow interviewed them, every single man had a college degree. Six had PhDs. There were six college professors in the group, an architect, a lawyer, an engineer, two ministers, four teachers, and a social worker. Behind the statistics, Crow found that almost every man had a fascinating life story to tell.

Max Kampelman had decided before the experiment was even over to hitch his wagon to Hubert Horatio Humphrey, the fastest-rising star in Minnesota politics. The two had first met at a professor's small apartment in Dinkytown, a university neighborhood densely populated with bookstores, coffee shops, and liberal faculty. Humphrey was just nine years older than Kampelman, but Kampelman readily looked to the newly elected mayor as a mentor. It was clear to the inner circle, of which Kampelman quickly became a member, that Humphrey's political ambitions and skill were equally grand. As for ideology, Kampelman was attracted by Humphrey's working class roots and his unapologetic liberalism. Humphrey liked Kampelman's intellect and tireless work ethic. While Kampelman continued his education and his teaching, he also became a trusted adviser to Humphrey. When Humphrey was elected to the U.S. Senate in 1948, the young Kampelman went with him to Washington to become Humphrey's sole legislative aide. Kampelman was twenty-eight.

In the postwar political foment of Minnesota, the liberal Humphrey actually found his most formidable political pressure on the left, from the Communists and the Socialists who were making a large impact in the state's labor unions and farmer cooperatives. As a Humphrey loyalist, Max began to develop into an enthusiastic anti-Communist. To Max, it was plain that the American Communists were pawns of the Soviet Union, and were trying to subvert labor solidarity and enlightened liberalism for the sake of Russian national interest. Max, Humphrey, and their loyalists tried at every turn to distance the American left from communism. One of Max's early books, *The Communist Party vs. the C.I.O.*, presented the battle in heroic terms, with American labor coming out on top over the sinister Reds. A deeply ingrained anti-Communism contributed to Humphrey's later refusal to disavow the Vietnam War, a stance that disappointed and puzzled many of his supporters, and may have cost him the presidency.

Max's anti-Communist ideology was also fueled by accounts of the Soviet treatment of Jews. While anti-Semites in the United States had long accused Jews and Communists of being one and the same, it was clear that anti-Semitism in the land of the pogrom had survived the Communist Revolution. Since 1948, the Soviets had been campaigning against the people it called "rootless cosmopolitans." In 1952, Stalin announced to the politburo, "every Jew is a nationalist and potential agent of the American intelligence." Stalin-era anti-Semitism climaxed with the so-called Doctor's Plot in 1953, when hundreds of Soviet Jewish doctors were arrested under the pretense that they were trying to secretly poison the Soviet leadership. Many of those doctors were never seen again. While being an ardent anti-Communist was the strategically correct stance for a member of the Humphrey political operation, it was not a stance that Max had to fake. Max's zeal would become well known to the Soviets. Once while Kampelman was in the middle of arms negotiations with the Soviets, the Soviet propaganda paper *Isvestia* described Kampelman's "cheap posturing," and his "zoological hatred for Communism."

Max had renounced his pacifism in 1945 when the atomic bomb fell on Hiroshima. The years following only solidified his feeling that pacifism was not a realistic option in the Cold War world. As a young man, he had joined the CPS as a clear demonstration of his pacifist beliefs. In 1955, he made an equally clear gesture to renounce them. He joined the Marine Corps Reserve. At thirty-four, and with his many government commitments, it was a largely symbolic gesture, but it spoke volumes about the philosophical distance he had traveled since his days in the Jewish Peace Fellowship.

Kampelman, while steadily building up his own law practice and network of contacts, remained a trusted friend and aide to Humphrey throughout his career, through his first stint in the Senate (1949–1965), his vice presidency to Lyndon Johnson (1965–1969), and his return to the Senate from 1971 until Humphrey's death from bladder cancer in 1978. At the heels of a master, Kampelman learned the art of politics and made a variety of friends in powerful places.

In 1980, President Carter, in the final months of his administration, asked Kampelman to represent the United States at the Conference on Security and Cooperation in Europe in Madrid. The conference was part of an ongoing discussion with the Soviets that was becoming increasingly important as Cold War tensions escalated. Kampelman was the ideal man for the job. While he was philosophically a well-known and ardent anti-Communist, he had great personal charm and a real ability to get along with almost anybody, a characteristic Max and all the other volunteers had been carefully screened for back in 1944. Starting with the talks in

Madrid, Kampelman began his second career of going "jaw to jaw" with the Soviets. He would stay on the job for incoming president Ronald Reagan, eventually becoming an ambassador and head negotiator to the START talks in Geneva in 1985, and counselor at the summit in Reykjavik, Iceland, in 1986. It was the perfect role for a man who had lost his pacifism in the blinding flash of the atomic bomb blast at Hiroshima—he was now charged with reducing the nuclear arms stockpiles of the world.

Everyone on all sides of the political spectrum recognized Max's great natural talent as a negotiator. The *Times* of London wrote after the successful conclusion of the Geneva talks, "The achievement is very much Kampelman's own. In many ways, he is the perfect negotiator—patient, cunning, and unfailingly courteous."

The public recognition of Max's work would culminate with the nation's highest civilian honor, the Presidential Medal of Freedom, in 1999. President Bill Clinton awarded Kampelman the medal in the East Room of the White House. He lauded Kampelman for his long diplomatic career—but also began his remarks with a mention of the starvation experiment.

"Max Kampelman," President Clinton said, "was probably not the first young man to work his way through college who made ends meet by skipping meals."

Max Kampelman was not the only guinea pig to leave Minnesota with an above average inclination to persevere and succeed. Roscoe Hinkle earned a PhD in sociology and became a professor at Ohio State University. While he would leave the Church of the Brethren, he remained a lifelong pacifist. Carlyle Frederick felt a strong pull to return to his rural home in Nappanee, Indiana. While Frederick became a schoolteacher, he built a home on what had been his ancestral family farm.

Robert Willoughby became a junior high school social studies teacher, but even decades later was still stung by the cheating accusation leveled at him by Dr. Keys. The sting was tempered somewhat by the fact that his fellow volunteers universally believed Willoughby when he said that he never veered from the diet.

Lester Glick celebrated his emancipation from the lab in 1945 by ignoring the strong recommendations of the doctors who had watched his every move for the last year. He would not report to a tuberculosis sanitarium. He had spent enough time away from his hilly family farm at Sugar Creek, Ohio, and he had the unscientific conviction that his own family might be able to take better care of him than strangers in a hospital. His mother, he wrote, "had always been successful in satisfying my nutritional needs." Her regimen of smothering attention combined with equally impressive servings of fried rabbit, pudding meat, ham, and sweet potatoes proved to be the perfect rehabilitative diet for a young man suffering from both starvation and tuberculosis. In spite of the doctors' misgivings, Lester gained 79 pounds in six months at home and fully recovered from TB.

Harold Guetzkow, the CPS man who worked on Keys' staff, invented an entirely new academic field in his poststarvation career. As the Cold War dawned in the 1950s, Guetzkow became concerned that global nuclear war might become inevitable. He began to develop complex models to simulate international decision-making processes, for the first time applying Game Theory to the social sciences. He retired as a full professor at Northwestern University in 1985, and received numerous awards for his unique contribution to the study and prevention of conflict. When asked what effect working with Keys might have had on his career, he said, "I learned to think big."

Jasper Garner, who had attended the same missionary school in India as Henry Scholberg, became a biologist, and was still working for the EPA in 2004 at the age of eighty-three. George Ebeling, the actor who sometimes annoyed his comrades with his dramatics in Shevlin Hall, managed to carve out a solid career as a character actor on stage and screen, appearing alongside James

Earl Jones in *The Great White Hope*. After the dinners at Shevlin Hall, he was inured to even the toughest critics. Unlike Max Kampelman, most of the test subjects maintained their pacifism throughout their lives. In some cases, that commitment to peace only deepened with time.

On January 18, 2003, Washington, D.C., hosted its largest anti-war rally since Vietnam, as the United States prepared to invade Iraq. Organizers estimated the crowd at two hundred thousand. The freezing temperatures kept heavy coats on and T-shirt slogans mostly hidden, but everyone, it seemed, carried a sign blasting the forty-third president, George W. Bush. The rally contained the usual cast of characters for a modern protest: shrill college kids, earnest academic liberals, worrisome anarchists, and aging baby boomers for whom protest was an act of nostalgia. A man in a rubber Bush mask with tape over its mouth vied for attention with an Uncle Sam on stilts carefully stepping his way through the crowd.

Despite the colorful assortment of protestors eager to talk to the press, at least one reporter was intrigued by a quiet, graying man who looked both entirely too old and too sick to be spending a freezing January morning on the march. She approached him. "I wouldn't let a cold stop me," he said, blowing his nose. "I've just had to bring a bucket of tissues with me." The protestor was eighty-six-year-old Sam Legg.

Sam Legg left Minneapolis with the most visible and lasting reminder of the experiment—his maimed left hand. His only complete fingers on that hand were his thumb and his pinky. He adapted quickly, and even learned to type with both hands, although he found that his pounding method worked best on the less-sensitive manual typewriters. For years, Sam maintained that the incident had been accidental, even believing that himself. Gradually, though, he came to realize and accept the huge psychological toll the experiment had taken on him, and the possibility that the swing of that ax may have been intentional. Sam learned later that the kind elderly ladies who had hosted that fateful dinner had actually conducted a burial ceremony for his severed fingers in their backyard.

Within a few short years of the experiment, Sam Legg was a Quaker. While he had become a CO and joined the CPS as an Episcopalian, he had learned much about the Friends in the CPS camps and after. Quaker doctrine, it seemed, with its emphasis on pacifism and a personal experience of the divine, seemed to match comfortably the religious philosophy Sam had come to on his own. Sam began a career in education after the experiment. By the time he became headmaster at a Quaker high school in Sandy Springs, Maryland, he had long since formalized his connections with the Quaker church. Never one to adopt a philosophy half-heartedly, Sam began volunteering to work with the American Friends Service Committee, both at home and abroad. With his knowledge of the language, he became a valuable asset on many AFSC missions to France.

Sam moved from the high school in Sandy Springs to Morgan State, a historically black college in Baltimore. He was hired as an adviser to foreign students, but was quickly promoted to director of admissions. Because of his many able years of service at Morgan State, only Sam thought it odd to be a white man in that position at a black college.

At Morgan State, Sam was able to witness—and support—some of the most turbulent years of the black power movement. He was also able to attend anti–Vietnam War rallies in nearby Washington, D.C., where he was frequently arrested and carted away during choreographed displays of civil disobedience. Although he retired from Morgan State in 1975, his relationship with the Washington police continued. On June 3, 1999, at the age of eighty-two, Sam was arrested as part of a group protesting President Clinton's bombing of Yugoslavia.

In 2005, Sam lives in an apartment in Broadmead, a Quaker retirement community located in the Hunt Valley near Baltimore. Just down the road in that same community is the home of Marshall Sutton, the young man with whom he shared the drive to Minneapolis in Sam's Packard in 1944. The old friends still discuss Quaker theology and the adventures in their future.

Lewis Hershey, the general who had been instrumental in forming the Civilian Public Service at the dawn of World War II, would continue to be a strong behind-the-scenes advocate for objectors as the war wound down. As early as VE day in May 1945, Hershey began advocating a point system that would allow CPS men to return to civilian life based on length of service, age, dependents, and other mitigating factors—a system nearly identical to that used for discharging soldiers. Political reality made it impossible for Hershey to treat objectors the same as military personnel. Despite Hershey's sympathy for the unpaid, sincere men in the camps, the CPS would survive until well past the end of the war. The system, in fact, would not discharge its last CO until March 31, 1947.

By the start of the Korean War in 1950, the camp system that was so central to the CPS had been scrapped. Objectors now participated in the 1-W system, where they were assigned on an individual basis to various service jobs, mostly in hospitals. From 1952 to 1955, more than ten thousand conscientious objectors would participate in this program, a program that was widely seen as acceptable to the peace churches and an improvement on the CPS.

Hershey retired as head of the Selective Service on February 16, 1970, after serving six presidents over twenty-nine years in that position, and an astonishing fifty-nine years in the military. As the domestic debate over the Vietnam War raged, protestors often held up the aging Hershey as an emblem of a corrupt system that supported an immoral war. For religious conscientious objectors, though, the long, sympathetic tenure of the general with pacifist ancestors had been a blessing.

The legal definition of a conscientious objector continued to evolve. The World War I law had required objectors to be from specific, recognized pacifist sects. The 1940 act, the act that created the CPS, had broadened the description to include those who had come to their pacifism "by reason of religious training or belief." Thus, a pacifist like Max Kampelman, not from one of the traditional peace churches, could be legally recognized. Some felt that description too broad, and too difficult for local boards to interpret. In 1948 the definition was narrowed somewhat, requiring a belief in a "Supreme Being." In 1965, the Supreme Court declared the Supreme Being clause unconstitutional, and the law was broadened once again to include anyone who "by reason of religious training and belief, is conscientiously opposed to participation in war in any form." The current definition is broadened even further, allowing objection based on moral as well as religious principles—modern COs need not belong to any religion at all.

With the expanding definition and the expanding resistance to the war, applications for CO status rose steadily throughout the Vietnam War era. During World War II, a scant .15 percent of inductees became conscientious objectors. As Hershey predicted, their tiny numbers made it possible and desirable for the military to do without them. The percentage of draftees applying for CO status during Vietnam mirrored the growing opposition to the war. The figures are 8.5 percent in 1968, 13.5 percent in 1969, 25.6 percent in 1970, and 42.6 percent in 1971. Astonishingly, by 1972, an actual majority of draftees were classified as COs—57 percent. In that year 33,041 men were classified as COs, almost three times as many as were in the CPS for the duration of World War II. Facing political crisis, President Nixon attempted to bolster his popularity and reduce opposition to the war by killing the unpopular system that General Hershey had carefully crafted over three decades. The result was an all-volunteer military. No American has been drafted since June 30, 1973.

With the advent of the all-volunteer force, defining conscientious objection has become a less urgent matter. Occasionally a soldier or sailor will decide in mid-tour that he can no longer morally carry arms. He must then initiate a long, meandering process that is in keeping with the best traditions of military bureaucracy. If the process doesn't outlast the objector's enlistment contract, he has a tough case to prove: the case that he or she is deeply, morally opposed to war, despite volunteering for the military, generally in the recent past. The cumbersome process has its advantages. Since there are numerous easier ways out of the military, the system ensures that those who follow the CO route to its conclusion are probably sincere.

The football stadium's memorial arch is again on display. Rescued from demolition by the class of 1942, it languished in pieces for years in dusty warehouses, almost forgotten. When the McNamara Alumni Center was constructed on the site of the old stadium in 2000, the old memorial arch once again saw the light of day. The Heritage Gallery is a museum inside the center devoted to University of Minnesota history and nostalgia. Among the predictable sports memorabilia is a wall of more than five thousand books relating to the university. Both volumes of *The Biology of Human Starvation* are present. The entrance to the gallery is the memorial arch, looking awkward and out of place in its modern surroundings. The arch is now tilted forward at a fifteen degree angle, in an attempt to make it fit in with the modern, angular aesthetic. The once straightforward memorial to the war dead seems uncomfortable with its new look, a look that comes dangerously close to parody.

On October 20, 1945, the experiment was over. The war was over. But Henry Scholberg was still in the CPS. No one seemed to know exactly when his time would be up, so Henry began looking for another assignment, another project where he might put his pacifist beliefs into action.

He found what he was looking for in a CPS bulletin asking for "sea-going cowboys." The United Nations Relief and Rehabilitation Administration was taking livestock to Europe by the shipload, hoping to get food on the hoof directly to the people, so they might be able to restart farming and husbandry. While the starvation experiment had been a painful exercise in expanding the body of scientific knowledge in a way that would theoretically aid the hungry, here was a chance to actually deliver nourishment to the starving victims of war. As if that wasn't enough, the agency was going to pay the cowboys $150 a trip—serious money in those days, especially when compared to the $5 a month Henry had gotten by on in the CPS. Henry eagerly filled out the application.

Neither his eagerness nor his experience with starvation did much to dampen his ingrained smart-ass tendencies. The application asked if he had any farm experience—Henry wrote that he had a "nodding acquaintance with cows." Few men, however, were volunteering to go overseas—millions were trying to come home. So the UN accepted Henry into the program despite his thin credentials. Henry boarded a converted Liberty ship in Newport News, Virginia. Soon, he, a handful of other cowboys, and several hundred head of cattle were en route to Gdansk, Poland.

The trip was exhilarating to Henry, as he reveled in the ship's mess, food that the rest of the crew found bland. His weight climbed slowly, but his energy soared, far beyond the level required for the small amount of work assigned to him: shoveling a large amount of soiled straw overboard in the morning and replacing it with a fresh supply. Henry made friends, discussed his pacifism with the curious crew, and read every page of *War and Peace.*

Near the end of the voyage, Scholberg's ship eased into the Kiel Canal to avoid the lengthy and potentially stormy trip around Jutland. As they plodded slowly through the sixty-mile-long canal, at times almost seeming to scrape the land on both sides, Henry got his first look at the war.

No building seemed to have survived intact. Everywhere there were craters, collapsed walls, and burned out tanks and jeeps. Allied vehicles zipped up and down the roads that paralleled the canal as if part of an ongoing victory proclamation. The adults they saw, almost all of them elderly, would barely glance at them, in a way that made it impossible to tell if they were bitter Germans in defeat or allies exhausted in their liberation. In contrast, the children were unabashedly happy to see them. Occasionally kids would race down the banks, yelling in German and clapping their hands for them to throw food. One day Henry brought a small sack of oranges topside; he threw them one at a time onto the bank, causing a commotion with each throw. When his arm wore out, a few of the oranges landed short, but the children jumped in the water to retrieve them. The kids looked seven or eight years old; it occurred to Henry that they had probably never seen an orange before. They had lived their whole lives in war.

Henry made two round trips to Poland on the cattle ships before finally being mustered out of the CPS. He moved back to Minnesota, the land of his ancestors and the place he had lived the longest outside of India. He charted a brief course in journalism, moved into teaching, and remained active in liberal politics. While Henry's stage was never as national as Max's, he was a Humphrey advocate in Minnesota, and was even elected as the Anoka County DFL party chairman in 1956. He married Phyllis Nelson in 1951, started having beautiful children, and seemed on course to become a successful small town politician.

By 1957, Henry was confident enough in his connections and

his reputation to run for mayor of Columbia Heights, the working class Minneapolis suburb in which he lived. Henry qualified for the general election in the primary. He seemed to be headed for the mayor's office, when the whispering campaign began.

Henry had made no attempt to hide what he had done during the war, but he didn't go out of his way to tell people about it either. His opponent did. The whispers about Henry's CO status became so strong that Henry felt compelled to respond with a flier four days before the election. "Scholberg's War Record," read the headline.

> A *whispering campaign has been going the past few weeks about Henry Scholberg and his activities during the World War II period.*
> *Let us look at the record:*
> *Henry Scholberg was inducted into the service just as 13 million other young men were during the war. There was only one factor of difference. Henry Scholberg had very strong convictions against killing.*

The flyer went on to detail Henry's work during his years in the CPS. It wasn't enough. Memories of the war were still fresh for many in 1957. Even in liberal Minnesota, voters were reluctant to elect a man who had opted out, no matter how sincere or virtuous his reasons. Henry lost the election by 64 votes.

On the night he lost the election, Henry was thirty-six years old. He realized then that he never wanted to run for elected office again. To solidify that choice, he drank a can of beer on his front porch for the whole world to see, an act nearly as objectionable to small town voters as conscientious objection. Teaching, Henry decided, was also not his calling. While enjoying the beer, he thought about what he might do next.

Like many of the starvation experiment guinea pigs, in the face of uncertainty Henry opted for further education. He obtained a master's degree in library science from the University of Minnesota. In 1961, he became the university's first curator of the Ames Library of South Asia, a massive collection donated to the university by a publishing scion. Once again, Henry's adulthood had been guided by his youth in India. He was the caretaker of thousands of books and maps that described the land of his birth, a land that he loved. Henry's literary output reflected his passion for cataloguing the literature of India. *The District Gazetteers of British India: A Bibliography* was published in 1970. He published a work in French, *Bibliographie des Français dans L'Inde* in 1973. Finally, he published what he called his "magnum opus" in 1982: *The Bibliography of Goa and the Portuguese in India.* Few people have ever been more happily matched in aptitude and vocation. Henry was curator of the Ames Library for twenty-five years.

Henry was alone among the volunteers in his return to the Minneapolis campus. He and Ancel Keys were colleagues. Although both men worked at the same campus until retirement, Scholberg never spoke to Keys in the days and years that followed the experiment. It was nothing intentional. Like most of the guinea pigs, Henry greatly respected Ancel Keys and was proud of having worked with him. Maybe it was the vast size of the Minneapolis campus that kept them apart, or perhaps the great academic distance between their two fields. Whatever the reasons, Henry never crossed paths with Keys during their careers at the University of Minnesota. Henry would, however, sometimes see the famous doctor in the distance, striding purposefully to his next lecture.

ACKNOWLEDGMENTS

————⟨◦⟩————

BEING MENTIONED in this section is wholly inadequate compensation for all these folks have done. Without them, there would be no book.

First, I wish to thank the starvation experiment volunteers who took the time to talk to me, welcome me into their homes, and in many cases give me documents and stories that contributed greatly to this text. The test subjects who helped are, in alphabetical order, William Anderson, Harold Blickenstaff, Carlyle Frederick, Jasper Garner, Earl Heckman, Roscoe Hinkle, Max Kampelman, Sam Legg, L. Wesley Miller, Richard Mundy, Henry Scholberg, Charles Smith, Marshall Sutton, and Robert Willoughby. Talking to you was not just a privilege—it was a lot of fun. Thank you again.

Ancel and Margaret Keys also welcomed me into their home, in Minneapolis, and provided me with invaluable documentation and incredibly interesting conversation. I regret that Dr. Keys did not live to see this book. I would have treasured his gruff, brutally honest, and powerfully insightful critique. May he rest in peace.

Dr. Henry Keys, Ancel's son, also took time out of his busy schedule to talk to me, as did Dr. Harold Guetzkow, Dr. Harry Blackburn, Dr. Scott Crow, and Dr. David Smith.

At the University of Minnesota Archives, Karen Klinkenberg deserves special mention for all her help. Karen repeatedly went above and beyond the call of duty to help me with this project, suggesting contacts and steering me toward the right people and places. Much of this book was written at the Christopher Center, at Valparaiso University, one of the finest university libraries in the nation.

Acknowledgments

Jill Langford published my first book, and she had a huge hand in helping this book see the light of the day by referring me to Frank Scatoni and Greg Dinkin of Venture Literary. With their skillful assistance, I was able to connect with Liz Stein of Free Press, for what has been the most rewarding relationship of my writing career. Maris Kreizman of Free Press was also a great help. Thank you all.

Now, two names that appeared in the acknowledgments section of my last book, and will I hope appear in all my future books: Doug Bennett of New Albany, Indiana, and Professor Tom Buchanan of the University of Tennessee at Chattanooga. All writers should have friends this good.

And finally, those family members who were good enough to read through rough drafts of this book and make invaluable suggestions: my parents, Ken and Laura Tucker, my sister Jennifer Tucker, and my wife, Susie Tucker, to whom this book is dedicated. My children, Colleen, Shannon, and Andrew, did not proofread or copyedit, but were a constant inspiration nonetheless.

NOTES

————⟨◇⟩————

Abbreviations

AMS Keys, Ancel. *Adventures of a Medical Scientist: Sixty Years of Research in Thirteen Countries*. Minneapolis: Ancel Keys, 1999. Copy provided to author by Dr. Keys.

BOHS Keys, Ancel, Josef Brozek, Austin Henschel, Olaf Mickelsen, and Henry Longstreet Taylor. *The Biology of Human Starvation*. 2 vols. Minneapolis: University of Minnesota Press, 1950.

ENW Kampelman, Max M. *Entering New Worlds: The Memoirs of a Private Man in Public Life*. New York: HarperCollins, 1991.

ESIM Keys, Ancel, Joesef Brozek, Austin Henschel, Olaf Mickelsen, and Henry Longstreet Taylor. *Experimental Starvation in Man*. Minneapolis: University of Minnesota Press, 1945. Provided to author by Carlyle Frederick.

MSJ *Minneapolis Star Journal*

Chapter 1: High Altitude Studies

8 *700 calories a day:* "War Stories: Lifting the Lid on the Siege of Leningrad," Wellcome News, Q1 2001, 27.

8 *473 calories a day; children, 423:* Ibid.

10 *Russia "is the No. 1 one problem":* "Men Starve in Minnesota," *Life*, July 30, 1945, 20.

11 *Lon Chaney wouldn't move to California:* Michael F. Blake, *Lon Chaney: The Man Behind the Thousand Faces* (Lanham, MD: The Vestal Press, 1990), 24. Lon did move to LA briefly with his cousin, Hugh Harbert, in 1904. By the time of the Great Earthquake, however, he appears to have moved to Oklahoma City and gotten married. In fact, his only child, Creighton Tull Chaney, was born on Feb. 10, 1906, in Oklahoma City, just two months before the earthquake.

11 *not a religious household:* AMS, 3.

12   *only 22 percent of the American population:* National Center for Educa-
     tion Statistics, *2000 Digest of Education Statistics: NCES 2001-034,*
     Table 8.
13   *two bowls of chow fan:* "The Fat of the Land," *Time,* January 13, 1961, 51.
13   *dried prunes:* Ibid.
13   *Needles, California:* AMS, 4.
16   *Dr. Paul Cadman:* William Hoffman, "Meet Monsieur Cholesterol," *Uni-
     versity of Minnesota Update* (Winter 1979). Available on www.mbbnet.
     umn.edu.
17   *The Weight-Length Relation in Fishes:* Ancel B. Keys, "The Weight-
     Length Relation in Fishes," *The Proceedings of the National Academy of
     Sciences,* vol. 14 No. 12, 922–925, December 1928. University of Min-
     nesota Archives.
18   Lon Chaney Is Dead: AMS, 9.
19   *"What do you propose to do in my lab?":* AMS, 11.
20   *"he had throat disease":* Ancel Keys, interview with author
20   *the lethality of hydrogen cyanide gas:* John B. West, *High Life: A History
     of High Altitude Physiology and Medicine* (New York: Oxford University
     Press for the American Physiological Society, 1998), 122.
21   *the radial artery of his left arm:* Ibid., 123.
21   *"impaired physical and mental powers":* Ibid., 128.
22   *90 out of a maximum 100 points:* Elsworth R. Buskirk, "Ancel Keys'
     Contributions to Physiological Hygiene." Speech given to the First Inter-
     national Keys Symposium on Nutrition and health, Minneapolis Hilton
     Hotel, Minneapolis, Minnesota, September 12, 2004, slide 36.
22   *full-blown fistfight:* West, *High Life,* 226. This is the only reference I
     could find to the fight between Forbes and Keys.
24   *seventeen scientific publications:* Ibid., 222.
24   *"real medical environment":* "The Fat of the Land," *Time,* January 13,
     1961, 51.
25   *"awfully provincial"* : William Hoffman, "Meet Monsieur Cholesterol,"
     University of Minnesota Update (Winter 1979).
25   *"to try to find out why people got sick before they got sick":* "The Fat of
     the Land," *Time,* January 13, 1961, 51.
26   *"the exact measurement of human function":* "Notes on the Laboratory
     of Physiological Hygiene, University of Minnesota, Minneapolis. Febru-
     ary 9, 1945," Ancel Keys Collection, University of Minnesota Archives, 3.
26   *"These are not questions of medicine or physiology":* Letter from Ancel
     Keys to Frank McCormick, December 7, 1945. Ancel Keys Collection,
     University of Minnesota Archives.
30   *"The letter K has no particular significance":* "Rations: Conference
     Notes," prepared by the Quartermaster School for the Quartermaster
     General, January 1949, 7. Accessible on the website of the Quartermaster
     Foundation, www.qmfound.com.
31   *a way to evaluate physical fitness in 1943:* Elsworth R. Buskirk, "Ancel
     Keys' Contributions to Physiological Hygiene," lecture given at the First

International Ancel Keys Symposium on Nutrition and Health, Sept. 12, 2004, Minneapolis MN, slide 15.

36 *fifty-five thousand dollars:* Joseph Blair, "Will You Starve that They be Better Fed?," 9. Brochure read at the Mennonite Historical Society, Goshen College, Goshen, Indiana.

Chapter 2: Work of National Importance

39 *"they will not 'shoot'":* War of the Rebellion, Official Records, Series I, Vol. XII, Part III, 835. Letter from Jackson to Col. S. Bassett French, March 21, 1862.

40 *"any well-recognized religious sect":* Heather Frazer and John O'Sullivan, *"We Have Just Begun to Not Fight": An Oral History of Conscientious Objectors in Civilian Public Service in World War II* (New York: Twayne Publishers, 1996), xiii.

40 *"I didn't want to go to war":* Alvin York, *York Diary,* from Alvin York Institute, available at http://volweb.utk.edu/Schools/York/diary.html.

40 *504 conscientious objectors:* Frazer, *"We Have Just Begun to Not Fight,"* xiv.

42 *34,506,923 American men:* Albert N. Keim, *The CPS Story: An Illustrated History of Civilian Public Service* (Intercourse, PA: Good Books, 1990), 8.

43 *his father's dramatic split from the River Brethren:* Roscoe Hinkle, interview with author.

44 *4,665 Mennonite, 1,353 Brethren, and only 951 Friends:* Melvin Gingerich, *Service for Peace: A History of Mennonite Civilian Public Service* (Akron, PA: The Mennonite Central Committee, 1949), 452. Other religions on the list include Theosophists, Essenes, Christadelphians, and Doukhobors.

45 *fewer than 10 percent went into the CPS:* Merlin C. Shull, "Ministry to Servicemen: A Classification, 1945." Survey data provided reluctantly to author by Dr. Roscoe Hinkle. As a sociologist, he was loath to give me unpublished, uncorroborated survey data that was over fifty years old. Everyone seems to agree, though, with the survey's conclusion that the percentage of Brethren who chose to ignore their church's position and go into the military was surprisingly high.

45 *Even the Mennonites:* Gingerich, *Service for Peace,* 90.

45 *"Mennonite General":* Keim, *The CPS Story,* 24.

46 *"made work, and we were made to work it":* Henry Scholberg, *That's India: The Memoirs of an Old India Hand* (New Delhi: Bibliophile South Asia, 2002), 71.

46 *lice-infested underwear:* Keim, *The CPS Story,* 75–76.

47 *"was like growing up Finnish in Helsinki":* ENW, 9.

47 *lowest return rate of any major group:* Roger Daniels, *Coming to America: A History of Immigration and Ethnicity in American Life* (New York: HarperCollins, 1990), 225. The Irish were in second place.

47   *"here is better"*: ENW, 10.

48   *"Statement of Purposes"*: Statement of Purposes of the Jewish Peace Fellowship, undated, Max Kampelman papers, Minnesota Historical Society.

49   *Most Ambitious*: ENW, 28.

50   *"We'll never get anywhere for peace"*: ENW, 46.

50   *"little groups of neighbors"*: James W. Davis Jr. and Kenneth M. Dolbeare, *Little Groups of Neighbors: The Selective Service System* (Chicago: Markham Publishing Group, 1968), 57.

51   *DSS-47:* "Sample Form 47: Special Form for Conscientious Objectors," read at the Mennonite Historical Library, Goshen College, Goshen, Indiana.

52   *"Selective Service prefers"*: ENW, 44.

52   *"We will be in a favorable position for such efforts"*: Speech given to the War Resister's League, May 27, 1944. Text of speech in Max Kampelman collection at Minnesota Historical Society, 12.

53   *By the fall of 1943, one in six*: Gingerich, *Service for Peace,* 214.

54   *perfect Nazi salute*: Scholberg, *That's India,* 56.

55   *"just waiting"*: Ibid., 70.

56   *"was a member of a minority group"*: Ibid., 72.

56   *"inmates with keys"*: Keim, *The CPS Story,* 81.

59   *"I got to know a fellow named Jesus of Nazareth"*: Sam Legg, interview with author. Almost all of Sam's story has been obtained via interview.

59   *"a careful reading of the New Testament"*: Norman Thomas, *The Conscientious Objector in America* (New York: B.W. Huebsch, 1923), 30.

59   *"this House will in no circumstance"*: Robert Cohen, *When the Old Left was Young: Student Radicals and America's First Mass Student Movement, 1929–1941* (New York: Oxford University Press, 1993), 79.

59   *huge placard behind the speakers platform*: The specifics for the pledge ceremony are in large part borrowed from Thomas Merton's *Seven Storey Mountain*, which contains a wonderful, humorous description of the Oxford Pledge and student strike that took place while he was an undergraduate at Columbia in 1935. Thomas Merton, *The Seven Storey Mountain* (New York: Harcourt, Brace, and Company, 1948), 144–45.

59   *"support the government of the United States"*: Cohen, *When the Old Left was Young,* 90.

60   *39 percent of American college students*: Ibid., 80.

61   *The curriculum included*: Gingerich, *Service For Peace,* 307. Gingerich lists the specific outline for a Mennonite course, but I am assuming that the Quaker course was substantially the same.

62   *Congressman Joseph Starnes*: Frazer, "We Have Just Begun to Not Fight," xxi. Joseph Starnes and his amendment achieved a kind of mythical status among COs, a symbol of all the wasted potential of the CPS.

62   *German POWs*: Keim, *The CPS Story,* 97.

62   *In all, 1,500*: Frazer, "We Have Just Begun to Not Fight," xx.

62   *crushed in a feed grinder*: Gingerich, *Service For Peace,* 472. Gingerich lists the names and causes of death for all 14 men who died in Mennonite CPS camps.

Chapter Three: The Cornelius Rhoads Award

64 *"with the maintenance of controlled conditions"*: Joseph Blair, "Will you starve that they be better fed?" (Minneapolis: CPS Unit 115, 1944), 11. Brochure on file at the Mennonite Historical Society, Goshen College, Goshen, Indiana.

64 *"all the kooks"*: William Hoffman, "Meet Monsieur Cholesterol," *University of Minnesota Update* (Winter 1979), 4.

64 *four broad requirements*: BOHS, 64.

65 *"I am happy most of the time"*: BOHS, 1100.

65 *"reasonably clear-cut psychiatric syndromes"*: BOHS, 867.

65 *"a mess"*: BOHS, 901.

66 *"a personal sense of responsibility"*: BOHS, 64.

66 *"intimately related to the nutritional state"*: BOHS, 1040.

67 *the rich store of scientific mythology,"*: BOHS, 106.

67 *"overburdened with far more conclusions than facts,"*: BOHS, 1051.

68 *25.5 years old*: BOHS, 66.

68 *152.7 pounds*: BOHS, 66.

68 *169.6 pounds*: "Who's Average?" *Healthy Weight Journal*, Jan./Feb. 1998, Vol. 12, Issue 1, 3. There is, of course, some controversy about what exactly is the average weight of an American male, but most sources put it somewhere near this number.

68 *one year of college*: BOHS, 67.

68 *CAVD—426*: BOHS, 67.

68 *two complete standard deviations*: BOHS, 68.

68 *"cultural activities"*: BOHS, 868.

69 *11 percent of the CPS*: Albert N. Keim, *The CPS Story: An Illustrated History of Civilian Public Service* (Intercourse, PA: Good Books, 1990), 81. The Brethren accounted for 1,353 men out of 11,996.

69 *nine men out of thirty-six*: The nine Brethren volunteers were Dan Miller, Roscoe Hinkle, Jasper Garner, Carlyle Frederick, Wendell Burrous, Harold Blickenstaff, Raymond Summers, Earl Heckman, and Robert Willoughby.

69 *fellow Methodists*: The five Methodists were L. Wesley Miller, Woodrow Rainwater, William Anderson, Henry Scholberg, and Robert McCullagh. The five Friends were Marshall Sutton, Howard Lutz, William Stanton, James Graham, and Daniel Peacock.

69 *4,665 men*: Keim, *The CPS Story*, 81.

69 *"almost all of the other subjects"*: AMS, 35.

70 *mortality rate of 2 percent*: *Experiments and Research with Humans: Values in Conflict* (Washington, DC: The National Academy of Sciences), 18.

71 *The mortality rate ranged from 40 percent*: "General info on Major Walter Reed," www.wramc.amedd.army.mil/welcome.history.

71 *"the dirtiest, laziest, most degenerate"*: Douglass Starr, "Revisiting a 1930s Scandal, AACR to Rename a Prize," *Science*, 4/25/2003, Vol. 300, issue 5619, 573.

73 *"perhaps the most utterly repulsive"*: Telford Taylor, Opening Statement of the Prosecution. Reprinted in George J. Annas and Michael A. Grodin, *The Nazi Doctors and the Nuremberg Code: Human Rights in Human Experimentation* (New York: Oxford University Press, 1992), 84.

74 *personally approved by General Douglas MacArthur*: Peter Williams and David Wallace, *Unit 731: Japan's Secret Biological Warfare in World War II* (New York: The Free Press, 1989), 133.

74 *maruta*: Ibid., 36.

75 *Dr. Kazu Tabei*: Ibid., 237.

75 *Dr. Hisato Yoshimura*: Ibid., 238.

75 *Ryoichi Naito*: Ibid., 241.

Chapter 4: Control

79 *Civilian Public Service Unit 115*: photograph of sign in "Research for Relief," Elgin, IL: The Brethren Service Committee, 1945. Pamphlet read at the Mennonite Historical Society, Goshen College, Goshen, Indiana.

81 LET EVERY MAN PROVE HIS OWN WORK: Picture of sign is from pamphlet "Research and Relief." Two Bible quotes are Gal. 6:4 and 1 Cor. 27.

82 *"We are here because of the problem of relief feeding in general"*: Speech is derived from Keys' section of pamphlet "Research and Relief," 3–4.

83 *averaged 152.7 pounds*: BOHS, 66.

83 *Calculating the amount of fat*: BOHS, 175, Table 89.

84 *The sperm analysis was emblematic*: BOHS, 1089–90.

86 *A typical lunch*: BOHS, 1212.

87 *Jay had even gone to the same English-language school*: Jasper H.B. "Jay" Garner, "India and After," written on the occasion of the 60th anniversary of his graduation from Woodstock School, 5. Provided to author by Jay Garner.

87 *gourds tied around his arms*: Ibid.

87 *The elder Blickenstaff*: Harold Blickenstaff, interview with author.

87 *twelve-mile round trip*: Scholberg, *That's India*, 78.

88 *median induction date*: Induction date from each volunteer from Directory of Civilian Public Service. Calculation of median by author.

89 *"Minnesotans are inclined to work things out"*: ENW, 54.

90 *"push yourself to the absolute limit"*: BOHS, 723.

91 *Max's name*: 44: ESIM, 45.

93 *"Allied military authorities directing the battle"*: "German Attack Tears Holes in 1st Army Lines," MSJ, December 18, 1944, 1.

93 NAZI PUSH CALLED WORST ALLIED SETBACK SINCE '42: MSJ, December 21, 1944, 1.

93 *Minnesota draft boards would be taking a close look*: "Draft Boards to Comb Lists," MSJ, December 20, 1944, 13.

93 *Jay Garner's brother*: Jay Garner, interview with author.

95 *"Do you find yourself often sleepy"*: BOHS, 825.

95   *1.76 pounds each:* BOHS, 74.
95   *3,210 calories per day:* BOHS, 1212, Table 519.

Chapter Five: Crucifying the Flesh

96   *"as was the case during the 1941–42 siege of Leningrad":* BOHS, 106.
96   *1,570 calories per day:* BOHS, 74.
97   *SUPPER #2:* ESIM, 43. BOHS gives lists of ingredients, but ESIM actually lists how the foods were served.
98   *test tube full of vitamin C crystals:* AMS, 16.
98   *"Wow! My clothes look sloppy!":* Lester Glick, *My Legacy: Recollections of Family, Work, and Service* (North Port, FL: Lester and Doris Glick, 2000), read at the Mennonite Historical Library, Goshen College, Goshen, Indiana. The book includes a sizable excerpt from Glick's starvation diary. This quote is from the entry for March 16, 1945.
98   *"the time between meals has now become a burden":* Harold Steere Guetzkow and Paul Hoover Bowman, *Men and Hunger: A Psychological Manual for Relief Workers* (Elgin, IL: Brethren Publishing House, 1946), 19.
101   *"in the Orient":* BOHS, 785.
102   *"psychopathic":* BOHS, 886.
102   *"subject is a bisexual":* BOHS, 885.
102   *"beautiful friendship":* BOHS, 884.
103   *"run like hell":* Henry Scholberg, *That's India: The Memoirs of an Old India Hand* (New Delhi: Bibliophile South Asia, 2002), 79.
103   *trapped in the store's revolving door:* Jasper H.B. "Jay" Garner, "India and After," written on the occasion of the 60th anniversary of his graduation from Woodstock School, 7. Provided to author by Jay Garner.
103   *21 percent reduction in strength:* ESIM, 46. Average amount lifted dropped from 168.6 kg to 132.7 kg.
104   *5 feet 10 inches:* ESIM, 45. Converted from centimeters.
104   *142.34 pounds:* ESIM, 45. Converted from kilograms.
104   *pounding feet, swaying:* Keys comments on the changing nature of the collapse in ESIM, 32.
105   *106 seconds:* interpolated from a score of 32 given in ESIM, 45.
105   *"The picture is one of pure muscular weakness":* ESIM, 32.
106   FRENCH FOOD CRISIS GROWS MORE CRITICAL: Helen Kirkpatrick, MSJ, February 26, 1945, 2.
106   ENOUGH FOOD DOESN'T EXIST: Mark McGaffin, MSJ, April 4, 1945, 3.
106   *"Food is Key to Politics in Italy":* Clare Boothe Luce, MSJ, April 11, 1945, 21.
107   STARVATION RIDDEN HOLLAND: Helen Kirkpatrick, MSJ, April 12, 1945, 1.
107   *the A&P advertised:* MSJ, March 15, 1945, 5.
107   *four-part series:* Ovid A. Martin, "The Food Shortage: '44 Optimism Cause of Slim Diets in '45," MSJ, March 20, 1945, 2.

108 *24 pounds of sugar per year:* Amy Bentley, *Eating for Victory: Food Rationing and the Politics of Domesticity* (Urbana, IL: University of Illinois Press, 1998), 102.

108 *July 1945 survey:* Ibid., 103.

109 *The nation's powerful dairy lobby:* Richard R. Lingeman, *Don't You Know There's a War On? The American Home Front 1941–1945* (New York: G.P. Putnam's Sons, 1970), 275. The tax was ten cents per pound, and was widely hated. Even Eleanor Roosevelt lobbied for its repeal.

109 *boiled tongue, and stuffed beef heart:* Joanne Lamb Hayes, *Grandma's Wartime Kitchen: World War II and the Way We Cooked* (New York: St. Martin's Press, 2000). Heart is stuffed with onions, celery, and bread cubes, recipe is on 104.

110 *three-fifths of the population:* Bentley, *Eating for Victory,* 114.

110 *Four days later:* Marshall Sutton, *Semi-Starvation Diary,* entry for April 17, 1945. Provided to author by Marshall Sutton.

111 *April 19, 1945:* Marshall Sutton diary, April 19, 1945.

111 *the "fittest" of the group:* ESIM, 46.

111 *judged the strongest:* ESIM, 46.

111 *6 feet 3 inches and 182 pounds:* ESIM, 46, converted centimeters and kilograms.

112 *Plaugher's weight had stalled out at 156 pounds:* BOHS, 889. Weights and calorie totals for both Plaugher and Willoughby in this paragraph are interpolated from their weight loss graphs on this page.

113 *forty packs a day:* BOHS, 890.

113 *with a beer mug:* Jay Garner, letter to author dated June 17, 2004.

113 *A group of four:* Marshall Sutton diary, Feb. 16, 1945.

113 *Candida:* Ibid.

114 *"BUCHENWALD CAMP ATROCITIES":* MSJ, April 23, 1945, 1.

114 *forty-three thousand victims:* estimates of Holocaust deaths vary widely. This figure is from: Walter Laqueur, ed., *The Holocaust Encyclopedia,* (New Haven: Yale University Press, 2001) 97.

115 *"Where Life Is Cheap,":* MSJ, April 23, 1945, 1.

115 *Max complained about the effects:* BOHS, 882.

116 *"the power of love":* Max Kampelman, interview with author.

116 *"You saw I ate my own sandwiches":* Max Kampelman, speech delivered on March 3, 1945, before the Cosmopolitan Club at the University of Minnesota as part of program on "COs and World War II." Max Kampelman Collection, Minnesota Historical Society.

117 *"to preside over the liquidation of the British Empire."* Yogesh Chadha, *Gandhi: A Life* (New York: John Wiley and Sons, 1997), 384.

118 *small amount of lime juice:* Ibid., 391–92

118 *"miserable little old man":* Ibid., 388.

118 *"various fasting antics":* Ibid., 390.

118 *109 pounds to 91 pounds:* Ibid. 388.

118 *three million people:* Amartya Sen, *Poverty and Famines: An Essay on Entitlement and Deprivation* (New York: Oxford University Press, 1981),

52. There is some argument about the exact scope of the tragedy in Bengal, but Sen argues convincingly for this number.

119 *political blackmail:* Chadha, *Gandhi,* 388.

119 *"My religion teaches me that":* R.K. Prabhu and U.R. Rao, eds., *The Mind of Mahatma Gandhi* (Ahmedabad, India: Navajivan Publishing House: 1967), 34.

119 *"A genuine fast cleanses the body":* Ibid., 35

119 *"I believe there is no prayer":* Ibid., 35.

120 *John the Hermit in the Egyptian desert:* Teresa M. Shaw, *The Burden of the Flesh: Fasting and Sexuality in Early Christianity* (Minneapolis: Augsburg Fortress Publishers, 1998), 12.

120 *Antony, ate only a meal of bread, salt, and water once per day:* Ibid., 13.

121 *reduced sexual desires:* Ibid., 16–17.

121 *"conquering the body":* Rudolph M. Bell, *Holy Anorexia* (Chicago: University of Chicago Press, 1985), 52.

123 *"half won":* "War Only Half Won, Truman Asserts," MSJ, May 8, 1945, 1.

125 *from 6.6 on average during the control period to 15.1 at S12:* ESIM, 48.

125 *At S12, the men ranked "Appetite" with the biggest increase:* BOHS, 822.

126 *The meal they selected:* BOHS, 1215.

127 *"Small cheer and great welcome makes a merry feast":* Shakespeare, *The Comedy of Errors,* Act 3, scene 1.

127 *and orange peel:* Henry Scholberg, interview with author.

Chapter 6: The Stigmata of Starvation

128 *CPS Camp 116: Directory of the Civilian Public Service* (Washington, DC: The National Interreligious Service Board for Conscientious Objectors), 431.

128 *"even when I handle food":* BOHS, 887.

128 *"To do that which is right in the sight":* BOHS, 887.

129 *"such an individual must be singularly resistant:* BOHS, 888.

131 *One volunteer, Carlyle Frederick:* Carlyle Frederick, interview with author.

132 *1.33 quarts of urine per day:* BOHS, 671, Table 310, converted from cc.

132 *"of obscure etiology":* BOHS, 887.

132 *"Sense of failure was almost predominant":* BOHS, 887.

133 *"a buck-toothed, near-sighted caricature labeled 'Nip'":* MSJ, July 11, 1945, editorial page.

133 *the lists of liberated prisoners:* See one example in MSJ, June 12, 1945, 15.

134 *almost 14 percent to about 5 percent:* BOHS, 175, Table 89.

135 *an average of 95.8°F:* BOHS, 1160, Table 470.

135 *just 35 beats per minute:* BOHS, 1174, Table 484.

137 *something of a scapegoat:* BOHS, 902. Ebeling's unpopularity is discussed in numerous documents connected to the experiment.

138 *"So sharp are hunger's teeth"*: William Shakespeare, *Pericles, Prince of Tyre,* Act I, scene iv.

138 *"Let's leave this town; for they are hare-brain'd slaves"*: William Shakespeare, *King Henry IV,* part I: I, ii.

139 *"Woe, alas!"*: Shakespeare, *Macbeth,* II, iii.

139 *"How many people have I hurt"*: Henry Scholberg, *That's India: The Memoirs of an Old India Hand* (New Delhi: Bibliophile South Asia, 2002), 81.

139 *"I am going crazy"*: BOHS, 903.

140 *"stigmata"*: BOHS, 14.

141 *On June 22, 1945:* Exact date is from the invaluable diary of Marshall Sutton. Many others remember the visit. Unfortunately, the POW's name has been lost.

142 *"Anyway, the first thing the Krauts did"*: Details of the story the visiting POW told are lost along with his name. These details are borrowed from a POW of Bad Orb told to a reporter in the MSJ, April 10, 1945, p. 21.

143 *fifty pounds:* Marshall Sutton Diary—he did remember the exact weight loss of the visiting POW, the only detail of the visit he records—a telling indication of Sutton's priorities at that time.

143 *"I recognize your deviant behavior"*: A line from the talk remembered by Henry Scholberg, interview with author.

143 *a solitary pea fell from Max's fork:* Lester Glick, *My Legacy: Recollections of Family, Work, and Service* (North Port, FL: Lester and Doris Glick, 2000), 66. Read at the Mennonite Historical Library, Goshen College, Goshen, Indiana. Glick refers to Max as "Our lawyer-to-be."

145 *"Most had gaunt pinched faces"*: Major Marvin B. Corlette, letter to Dr. Ancel Keys, August 18, 1945. Copy provided to author by Jasper Garner.

146 *a similar case in Illinois:* IN RE CLYDE WILSON SUMMERS, 325 U.S. 561 (1945), No. 205. Decided June 11, 1945.

146 *"the decision, you will note"*: Max Kampelman, letter to Hon. Birdie Amsterdam, May 21, 1946. Minnesota Historical Society, Max Kampelman Papers.

146 *"proved to be a highly reliable and conscientious"*: Ancel Keys, letter to the Committee on Character and Fitness, December 17, 1945. Minnesota Historical Society, Max Kampelman Papers.

147 *"By volunteering for this program"*: Hubert H. Humphrey, Letter to the Committee on Character and Fitness, April 9, 1946. Minnesota Historical Society, Max Kampelman Papers.

147 *the result stayed close to .69 millimeters:* BOHS, 1190, Table 500.

148 *improved by a full standard deviation:* BOHS, 685.

150 *"This thing has undressed us"*: BOHS, 903.

151 *That all changed on June 29:* Date of photography from Marshall Sutton Diary.

152 *"this is something like tests given fliers"*: "Men Starve in Minnesota," *Life,* July 30, 1945, 45.

153 *"He's been stuck at 121 pounds"*: Glick, *My Legacy,* 66.

153 *"114 pounds"*: Ibid., 65.

153 *"Two slices of bread and 20 grams of potatoes"*: Ibid., 66.

153 *"watermelon balls"*: Marshall Sutton Diary.

154 *fried pork tenderloin, fried rabbit, fried mush*: Glick, *My Legacy*, 31. Glick devotes an entire page to a loving essay on the meals of his youth entitled "Our Family Cuisine."

155 *"That," whispered Jim, "is God's prize creation"*: Entire episode is from Glick, *My Legacy*, 68.

156 *the 5 foot 10 inch Sam Legg weighed only 105.6 pounds*: ESIM, 45, Table V.

156 *Harvard Fitness Test on that same day*: BOHS, 894.

156 *"No man can ever equal the machine"*: Sam Legg, "Sonnet." Provided by Marshall Sutton.

157 *the crust of burnt macaroni*: Glick, *My Legacy*, 70.

158 *He collapsed in nineteen seconds*: ESIM, 45, Table V.

158 *the average drop of 72 percent*: ESIM, 46, Table V.

158 *The crying started as the men were taking his pulse*: BOHS, 894.

158 *"I have never been so ashamed of any performance"*: BOHS, 894.

159 *"Right now you weigh 136.4 pounds"*: ESIM, 46, Table V.

160 *"In summary, this subject's latent personality weaknesses"*: BOHS, 891.

160 *"probable breaking of the diet," indicated by "indirect but convincing evidence"*: BOHS, 891.

161 *"hopelessly unable to express himself"* : BOHS, 892.

161 *an average of 152.7 pounds to 115.6 pounds*: BOHS, 66.

161 *a third of a centimeter in height*: BOHS, 134, Table 48.

161 *by almost 500 cubic centimeters*: BOHS, 1154, Table 464.

161 *The heart that pumped that blood had shrunk by 17 percent*: BOHS, 204. Size of heart was calculated using X-rays.

161 *The average score at S24 was 2.3*: BOHS, 1200, Table 510.

Chapter Seven: Restricted Rehabilitation

166 *"an important Japanese Army base"*: MSJ, August 6, 1945, 1.

166 *ATOMIC BOMB HITTING JAPS, TRUMAN REVEALS*: MSJ, August 6, 1945, 1.

166 *"It is an atomic bomb"*: MSJ, August 6, 1945, 1.

166 *2,000 times heavier*: MSJ, August 6, 1945, 1.

166 *Sixty-five thousand people*: MSJ, August 6, 1945, 1.

166 *two billion dollars had been spent*: MSJ, August 6, 1945, 1.

166 *refused to believe that such destruction could be caused by a single bomb*: MSJ, August 7, 1945, 6.

166 *ALL LIVING THINGS SEARED TO DEATH*: MSJ, August 8, 1945, 1.

166 *the Japanese dead at 100,000*: MSJ, August 8, 1945, 1.

167 *word that the rationing of canned food*: MSJ, August 15, 1945, 1.

168 *These dark patches around the eyes*: BOHS, 242.

168 *fingernails were blue*: BOHS, 242.

168 *the corneas were unnaturally white*: ESIM, 23.

169 *Sam* knew *he was:* Sam was in fact in the second to lowest group.

169 *"My god, Margaret," he said. "I am torturing them":* Margaret Keys recounted this conversation when she spoke to one of the guinea pig reunions years later. It was recalled by several of the guinea pigs in attendance.

170 *seven men were holding up worse than Legg at S24:* BOHS, 1200, Table 510.

174 *The next evening, on August 29, 1945:* Diary of Marshall Sutton.

175 *a miserable one tenth of one pound:* BOHS, 1137, Table 450, Group Z. Converted from kilograms.

175 *regained only 6.5 pounds:* BOHS, 1137, Table 450, Group T. Converted from kilograms.

175 *less than one fifth:* BOHS, 1137, Table 450, Group T. This particular group's average weight loss from C12 to S24 was 15.42 kilograms, or 33.9 pounds.

175 *percentage of body fat:* BOHS, 179.

175 *4.2 beats per minute:* BOHS, 1174, Table 484.

176 *The next day was September 9, 1945:* Diary of Marshall Sutton.

178 *The next day, September 13, Keys reversed his earlier decision:* BOHS, 70, Table 16. On p. 838, Keys wrote that the buddy system was abolished "in the face of imminent wholesale violation."

178 *In a widely distributed pamphlet:* "He Served his Country During the War," Washington: National Service Board for Religious Objectors. Pamphlet provided by Mennonite Historical Society, Goshen College, Goshen, Indiana.

179 *Committee to End Slave Labor:* Pamphlet read at the Mennonite Historical Society, Goshen College, Goshen, Indiana.

180 *28 percent of the men:* BOHS, 825, Table 362.

180 *Forty-one percent:* BOHS, 824, Table 362.

181 *"Take a look at Subject 130," he said:* BOHS, 901–4.

182 *the average weight had risen to 129.2 pounds:* BOHS, 1138, Table 450. Converted from kilograms.

182 *on average about 10 percent less:* BOHS, 1138, Table 450. These men had gone from 67.51 kg at C12 to 52.09 kg at S24 to 60.91 kg at R12.

182 *Keys would say it was the most significant finding of the study:* Ancel Keys, interview with author.

183 *"There is at present in operation":* ESIM, 7.

183 *"The subjects in this study are all conscientious":* ESIM, 11.

183 *"The results of the rehabilitation studies":* ESIM, 41.

184 *"It is an unpardonable error":* Harold Steere Guetzkow, and Paul Hoover Bowman, *Men and Hunger: A Psychological Manual for Relief Workers* (Elgin, Illinois: Brethren Publishing House, 1946), 52.

184 *"Above all, do not require people":* Ibid., 57.

184 *"Unnecessary exhibitions of strength":* Ibid., 54.

184 *"relived adolescence":* Ibid., 44.

184 *"it is our wish that practical":* Ibid., 11.

185 *a list of twenty-nine different foods:* Lester Glick, *My Legacy: Recollections of Family, Work, and Service* (North Port, FL: Lester and Doris Glick, 2000), 74. Read at the Mennonite Historical Library, Goshen College, Goshen, Indiana. Diary entry for October 19, 1945.

186 *Glick realized that he was sitting alone:* Ibid., diary entry for October 20.

Chapter Eight: The Helsinki Declaration

188 *"murders, tortures, and other atrocities committed in the name of medical science":* George J. Annas and Michael A. Grodin, *The Nazi Doctors and the Nuremberg Code: Human Rights in Human Experimentation* (New York: Oxford University Press, 1992), 67. Taylor's entire opening statement is reproduced.

188 *only Karl Brandt declined:* Ibid., 106.

189 *"special responsibility":* Ibid., 97–100.

189 *science fight another enemy of society":* "Prison Malaria: Convicts Expose Themselves to Disease so Doctors Can Study it," *Life,* June 4, 1945, 43.

189 *"Their subjects eat all the same food, sleep the same hours, and are never far away":* Ibid.

190 *"just about as important":* Nathan F. Leopold, *Life Plus 99 Years* (Garden City, NJ: Doubleday & Company, 1958), 307.

190 *"the experiment is to be discontinued":* Annas, *The Nazi Doctors,* 125.

190 *"the person concerned":* Ibid., 127.

191 *Karl Brandt attempted to dodge:* Ibid., 106.

192 *an estimated 70 percent of girls ceased having their menstrual periods:* BOHS, 749.

192 *1895 autopsy of a sixteen-year-old girl:* BOHS, 99.

192 *"normal":* BOHS, 966.

192 *In German-occupied Greece:* BOHS, 758.

192 *the mortality rate of females rose by 73 percent:* BOHS, 758.

192 *men made up 89.5 percent of all deaths deemed "natural":* BOHS, 760.

192 *"traditional woman's attitude of self-sacrifice and resignation":* BOHS, 760.

192 *"Clearly, the whole question merits the closest scrutiny":* BOHS, 760.

193 *"the relatively high cost of providing special protein feedings":* BOHS, 1063–64.

193 *"We do not wish to qualify our conclusion":* BOHS, 1064.

193 *worse than had been believed possible":* BOHS, 599.

193 *"The vast majority of the famine victims:* BOHS, 599.

194 *"The Belsen patients considered stomach tubes":* BOHS, 600.

194 *"a cause for rejoicing":* BOHS, 1065.

194 *A seven-year famine in Egypt starting in 1708* B.C.*":* BOHS, 1248. Genesis 41 is listed as the source, and it is unclear how the exact date of 1708 B.C. was derived.

194 *Table 565:* BOHS, 1246.

194 *J. Penkethman's 1748 work:* BOHS, 1315.

194 *thirty-seven-page operating manual:* BOHS, 1305.

194 *"My admiration was tinted with only one regret":* BOHS, xvi.

194 *"We regret, of course, that this work was not published":* BOHS, xxvi.

196 Dr. Andrew Ivy, *the Nuremberg prosecution's expert witness:* Evelyne Shuster, "The Nuremberg code: Hippocratic ethics and human rights." *Lancet,* March 28, 1998, Vol. 351, Issue 9107, p. 974.

197 *over four thousand separate experiments:* Danielle Gordon, "The verdict: No harm, No foul," *Bulletin of the Atomic Scientists,* Jan./Feb. 1996, Vol. 52, Issue 1, p. 33.

197 *Fernald State School in Massachusetts:* Ibid.

197 *cancer patients at the University of Cincinnati:* David Egilman, Wes Wallace, and Cassandra Stubbs, "A little too much of the Buchenwald touch? Military radiation research at the University of Cincinnati, 1960-1972." *Accountability in Research: Policies & Quality Assurance.* Jan. 1998, Vol. 6, p. 63.

197 *Between 1945 and 1965, from 500,000 to 2.3 million:* Danielle Gordon. "The verdict: No harm, No foul," *Bulletin of the Atomic Scientists,* Jan./Feb. 1996, Vol. 52, Issue 1, p. 33.

197 *retarded children at the Willowbrook State School:* Bruce Gordon and Ernest Prentice, "Protection of Human Subjects in the United States: A Short History," *Journal of Public Health Management Practice,* 2000, Vol. 6, issue 6, p5

197 *researchers at the Brooklyn Jewish Chronic Disease Hospital:* Ibid.

197 *70 percent of approved drugs had:* Jonathan Moreno, "Goodbye to all that," *Hastings Center Report,* May/June 2001, Vol. 31, Issue 3, p. 9.

198 *"In the treatment of the sick person":* Annas, *The Nazi Doctors,* 332. The entire declaration is reproduced.

199 Dr. David Smith, *a psychologist at the University of Notre Dame:* Interview with author.

199 Dr. Henry Keys, *son of Ancel and a cancer researcher:* Interview with author.

200 *"Trying to make meaningful psychological changes with an anorexic patient":* David M. Garner, Kelly M. Vitousek and Kathleen M. Pike, "Cognitive-Behavioral Therapy for Anorexia Nervosa," *Handbook of Treatment for Eating Disorders* (New York: The Guilford Press, 1997), 103.

200 *"their eyes staring and looking wild":* Nathaniel Philbrick, *In the Heart of the Sea: The Tragedy of the Whaleship Essex* (New York: Viking, 2000), 171.

200 Gavan Daws in *Prisoners of the Japanese:* Gavan Daws, *Prisoners of the Japanese: POWS of World War II in the Pacific* (New York: William Morrow and Company, 1994), 256–59.

200 In The Mapmaker's Wife, *Robert Whitaker:* Robert Whitaker, *The Mapmakers Wife: A True Tale of Love, Murder, and Survival in the Amazon* (New York: Basic Books, 2004), 260–61.

Chapter Nine: The Cover of *Time*

201 *the leading cause of death in the United States since 1921:* David Brown, "Keys of Nutrition: When America was hungry to understand the science of diet, Ancel Keys stepped up to the plate," *Washington Post,* October 22, 2002, Page HE01.

201 *"an important and remarkable substance quite apart":* Ancel Keys and Margaret Keys, *Eat Well and Stay Well* (Garden City, NY: Doubleday, 1959), 58.

202 *Hastings State was a hospital for the insane:* AMS, 39.

202 *"Our dietary experiments could do no harm":* AMS, 39.

203 *Finns in lumber camps, Keys witnessed with amazement:* AMS, 69.

204 *cause of death was gelosia:* AMS, 84.

204 *a glass of olive oil:* AMS, 88.

201 *992 out of 10,000 deaths:* David Brown, "Keys of Nutrition: When America was hungry to understand the science of diet, Ancel Keys stepped up to the plate," *Washington Post,* October 22, 2002, Page HE01.

204 *just 9 out of 10,000:* Ibid.

204 *about 40 percent:* Ibid.

204 *a pack a day or more—43 percent in Japan, 30 percent in Crete:* Ibid.

205 *The "Keys Formula" is still in wide use today:* Henry Blackburn gave this version of the Keys Formula at a tribute to Keys in 2004:

$$\Delta C = 1.35 \, (2\Delta S - \Delta P) + 1.5 \Delta Z$$

ΔC = Change in blood cholesterol

ΔS = Change in Saturated Fat

ΔP = Change in polyunsaturated Fat

ΔZ= the square root of the change in dietary cholesterol

205 *"one of the most widely published":* P. J. Scott, "Clinically Integrated Studies in Pathology: Their Contribution to Atherosclerosis Research," *Pediatric Pathology and Molecular Medicine,* 2002, Vol. 21, p. 247.

205 *"I've got five thousand cases":* "The Fat of the Land," *Time,* January 13, 1961, 50.

206 *"If some countries can do without heart attacks":* Henry Blackburn, "Ancel Keys, Pioneer," Speech given to the First International Keys Symposium on Nutrition and Health, Minneapolis Hilton Hotel, Minneapolis, Minnesota, September 12, 2004.

206 *"It is a happy blending of":* Keys, *Eat Well and Stay Well,* 7.

207 *"a greasy or waxy substance:* Ibid, 58.

207 *"the condition produced by interference":* Ibid., 23.

207 *"This is an extreme case of adaptation":* Ibid., 76.

207 *"Some of these believe practically nothing":* Ibid., 5

207 *"who take second place to none in cookery"* Ibid., 102.

207 *The Chinese restaurant owners of America:* William Hoffman, "Meet Monsieur Cholesterol," *University of Minnesota Update,* Winter 1979.

208 *"The Fat of the Land":* Time, January 13, 1961, 48–52.

208 *In 1962, Keys organized a high-altitude study:* Hoffman, "Meet Monsieur Cholesterol."

209 *"Americans have Sunday dinner every day":* Keys, *Eat Well and Stay Well,* 19. Just one mention of one of Keys' favorite quotes.

209 *"by the North American habit of turning the stomach into the garbage disposal":* Hoffman, "Meet Monsieur Cholesterol." Another frequently quoted line from Keys.

209 *"Ancel Keys has a quick and brilliant mind":* Henry Blackburn, "Ancel Keys, Pioneer." Speech given at the First International Ancel Keys Symposium on Nutrition and Health, Sept. 12, 2004, Minneapolis Hilton Hotel, Minneapolis, Minnesota.

210 *In all, 12,763 men between the ages of forty and fifty-nine:* Daan Kromhout, "Findings and History of the Seven Countries Study," Speech given at the First International Ancel Keys Symposium on Nutrition and Health, Sept. 12, 2004, Minneapolis Hilton Hotel Minneapolis, Minnesota.

211 *Ancel used to hold up chicken bones at the dinner table:* Carrie D'Andrea and Henry Keys, "Family Greetings." Speech given at the First International Ancel Keys Symposium on Nutrition and Health, Sept. 12, 2004, Minneapolis Hilton Hotel, Minneapolis, Minnesota.

211 *"I could never be a bedside handshaker"* : Ibid.

211 *"How do you know when you've done any good?":* Ibid.

211 *His old eyes, he wrote later:* AMS, 109.

211 *"My room is filled with books I cannot read":* AMS, 129.

Chapter Ten: Unrestricted Rehabilitation

214 *on average 5,219 calories per day:* BOHS, 1132, Table 449.

214 *managed to consume 11,500 calories:* BOHS, 121, Figure 33.

215 *"The experiment increased my capacity to cope with adversity":* Lester Glick, *My Legacy: Recollections of Family, Work, and Service* (North Port, FL: Lester and Doris Glick, 2000), 76. Read at the Mennonite Historical Library, Goshen College, Goshen, Indiana.

215 *a love of macaroni and cheese:* Ibid., 78.

215 *Dr. Crow was able to locate 19 of the original 36 guinea pigs:* Scott J. Crow, "Science and Philosophy in the Starvation Studies." Address delivered at First International Ancel Keys Symposium on Nutrition and Health, Sept. 12, 2004, Minneapolis Hilton Hotel, Minneapolis, Minnesota, Slide 40.

215 *distorted body images:* Ibid., Slide 48.

215 *by an average of 27 pounds:* Ibid., Slide 50.

216 *only three of the men said they never again:* Ibid., Slide 53.

216 *every single man had a college degree:* Ibid., Slide 41.

217 *One of Max's early books:* Max Kampelman, *The Communist Party vs. The C.I.O.: A Study in Power Politics* (New York: Frederick A. Praeger, 1957).

217 *"rootless cosmopolitans"*: http://en.wikipedia.org/wiki/Doctors'_plot.

218 *"cheap posturing," and his "zoological hatred for Communism"*: ENW, 10.

219 *"jaw to jaw"*: ENW, 235.

219 *"The achievement is very much Kampelman's own"*: ENW, 368.

219 *"Max Kampelman," President Clinton said:* William Jefferson Clinton, "Remarks by the President and the First Lady During the Medal of Freedom Event," August 11, 1999, available on www.medaloffreedom.com.

220 *"had always been successful in satisfying my nutritional needs"*: Glick, *My Legacy*, 74.

220 *"I learned to think big"*: Harold Guetzkow, interview with author.

222 *"I wouldn't let a cold stop me"*: Luciana Lopez, "Maryland Activists Prepare to Rally for Peace, Counter-Rally for Patriotism," Capital News Service, January 17, 2003.

223 *at the age of eighty-two, Sam was arrested:* Max Obuszewski, "Friend among 26 arrested trying to deliver peace letter to U.S. President Clinton," American Friends Service Committee, June 8, 1999. Available on www.quaker.org/peaceweb/kovdc1.html.

223 *As early as VE day in May 1945:* George Q. Flynn, *Lewis B. Hershey, Mr. Selective Service* (Chapel Hill, NC: University of North Carolina Press, 1985), 132.

223 *would not discharge its last CO until March 31, 1947:* Heather Frazer and John O'Sullivan, *"We Have Just Begun to Not Fight": An Oral History of Conscientious Objectors in Civilian Public Service in World War II* (New York: Twayne Publishers, 1996), 245.

223 *From 1952 to 1955, more than ten thousand conscientious objectors:* http://www.swarthmore.edu/Library/peace/conscientiousobjection/co%20 website/pages/history.html.

224 *"Supreme Being"*: Joseph E. Capizzi, "Selective Conscientious Objection in the United States," *Journal of Church and State*, Spring 1996, Vol. 38, issue 2, 339.

224 *modern COs need not belong to any religion at all:* "Fast Facts: Conscientious Objection and Alternative Service," The Selective Service System.

224 *.15 percent of inductees became conscientious objectors:* Frazer, *"We Have Just Begun to Not Fight,"* 247.

224 *5 percent in 1968, 13.5 percent in 1969, 25.6 percent in 1970, and 42.6 percent in 1971:* Ibid.

224 *Astonishingly, by 1972, an actual majority of draftees:* Ibid.

226 *$150 a trip:* Henry Scholberg, *That's India: The Memoirs of an Old India Hand* (New Delhi: Bibliophile South Asia, 2002), 82.

226 *"nodding acquaintance with cows"*: Ibid.

228 *"Scholberg's War Record"*: Ibid., 121.

228 *64 votes:* Ibid., 123

SOURCES

Annas, George J., and Michael A. Grodin. *The Nazi Doctors and the Nuremberg Code: Human Rights in Human Experimentation*. New York: Oxford University Press, 1992.

Backstrand, Jeffrey R. "The History and Future of Food Fortification in the United States: A Public Health Perspective." *Nutrition Reviews*. January 2002. Vol. 60, No. 1: 15–26.

Bacon, Margaret. *The Quiet Rebels: The Story of the Quakers in America*. New York: Basic Books, 1969.

Bailey, Herbert. "They Starved Themselves for You." *Argosy*. March 1957. 25. Provided to author by Jasper Garner.

Bell, Rudolph M. *Holy Anorexia*. Chicago: University of Chicago Press, 1985.

Bentley, Amy. *Eating for Victory: Food Rationing and the Politics of Domesticity*. Urbana: University of Illinois Press, 1998.

Big Flats: CPS Camp 46, Big Flats NY. Handbook read at Mennonite Historical Library, Goshen College, Goshen, IN.

Blackburn, Henry. "Ancel Keys, Pioneer." Speech given to the First International Keys Symposium on Nutrition and Health, Minneapolis Hilton Hotel, Minneapolis, MN, September 12, 2004.

Blair, Joseph. *Will You Starve That They Be Better Fed?* Minneapolis: CPS Unit 115, 1944. Brochure read in the Mennonite Historical Library, Goshen College, Goshen, IN.

Blake, Michael F. *Lon Chaney: The Man Behind the Thousand Faces*. Lanham, MD: The Vestal Press, 1990.

Bob Goes to Camp. Washington, DC: National Service Board for Religious Objectors: 1945. Brochure read at the Mennonite Historical Library, Goshen College, Goshen, IN.

Bowman, Paul Haynes. *Handbook for Use at Camp Lagro, Lagro, Indiana*. Read at Mennonite Historical Library, Goshen College, Goshen, IN.

Brady, Tim. "Behind Gate 27." *Minnesota Medicine*. May 2003. 22–25.

Brown, David. "Keys of Nutrition: When America Was Hungry to Understand the Science of Diet, Ancel Keys Stepped up to the Plate." *Washington Post*, October 22, 2002, HE1.

Brozek, Josef. "Psychology of Human Starvation and Nutritional Rehabilitation." *The Scientific Monthly*. April 1950, Vol. LXX, No. 4: 270–74.

———. "Nutrition, Malnutrition, and Behavior." *Annual Review of Psychology*. 1978. Vol. 29: 157–77.

Buchanan, Roderick D. "On Not 'Giving Psychology Away'": The Minnesota

Multiphasic Personality Inventory and Public Controversy Over Testing in the 1960s." *History of Psychology.* August 2002. 284–309.

Buhle, Paul. "Halting McCarthyism: The Stamler Case in History." *Monthly Review: An Independent Socialist Magazine.* October 1999. Vol. 51, Issue 5: 44.

Bush, E. M. "Strike Continues at Big Flats." 1945. Memo read at Mennonite Historical Library, Goshen College, Goshen, IN.

Buskirk, Elsworth R. "Ancel Keys' Contributions to Physiological Hygiene." Speech given to the First International Keys Symposium on Nutrition and Health, Minneapolis Hilton Hotel, Minneapolis, MN. September 12, 2004.

Capizzi, Joseph E. "Selective Conscientious Objection in the United States." *Journal of Church and State.* Spring 1996. Vol. 38 Issue, 2: 339.

Chadha, Yogesh. *Gandhi: A Life.* New York: John Wiley and Sons, 1997.

Chapman, Carleton B. "About Ancel Keys." An address presented at the retirement dinner of Dr. Keys, Minneapolis, MN. December 3, 1971. Copy provided to author by Dr. Keys.

Cohen, Ben, and Maura Lerner. "U scientist who invented the K ration dies at 100." *Minneapolis Star Tribune,* November 23, 2004.

Cohen, Robert. *When the Old Left Was Young: Student Radicals and America's First Mass Student Movement, 1929–1941.* New York: Oxford University Press, 1993.

Conscience Compels Them: The story of America's religious objectors to participation in warfare, and what is happening to them while their country is at war. Pamphlet read at the Mennonite Historical Library, Goshen College, Goshen, IN.

Corlette, Marvin B. "Statement on Visit to Physiological Hygiene Laboratory." Letter to Ancel Keys, August 18, 1945. Copy provided to author by Jasper Garner.

"Cornelius Packard Rhoads." *Dictionary of American Biography,* Supplement 6: 1956–1960. American Council of Learned Societies, 1980. Reproduced in *Biography Resource Center.* Farmington Hills, MI: The Gale Group, 2004. http://galenet.galegroup.com/servlet/BioRC.

Crawford, DeLisle. *A Civilian Public Service Through Medical Research: Work of Voluntary Human Guinea Pigs in Saving Life and Improving Health.* Philadelphia: American Friends Service Committee, 1945.

Crow, Scott J. "Science and Philosophy in the Starvation Studies." Speech given to the First International Keys Symposium on Nutrition and Health, Minneapolis Hilton Hotel, Minneapolis, MN. September 12, 2004.

D'Andrea, Carrie, and Henry Keys. "Family Greetings." Speech given to the First International Keys Symposium on Nutrition and Health, Minneapolis Hilton Hotel, Minneapolis, MN. September 12, 2004.

Daniels, Roger. *Coming to America: A History of Immigration and Ethnicity in American Life.* New York: HarperCollins, 1990.

Davis, James W., Jr., and Kenneth M. Dolbeare. *Little Groups of Neighbors: The Selective Service System.* Chicago: Markham Publishing Group, 1968.

Davis, Joseph S. "Food in a World at War." *Harvard Business Review.* Winter 1941, Vol. 19, Issue 2: 133.

Sources

————. "The World's Food Position and Outlook." *Harvard Business Review.* Autumn 1942. Vol. 21, Issue 1: 43.

Daws, Gavan. *Prisoners of the Japanese: POWS of World War II in the Pacific.* New York: William Morrow and Company, 1994.

Directory of Civilian Public Service. Washington, DC: The National Interreligious Service Board for Conscientious Objectors, 1996.

Dorman, John. "The Hippocratic Oath." *Journal of American College Health.* September 1995. Vol. 44, Issue 2: 84.

Edgerton, Jay. "Hungry Men are DIFFERENT Men." *The Minneapolis Sunday Tribune,* June 4, 1950, 1. Provided to author by Carlyle Frederick.

Egilman, David, Wes Wallace, and Cassandra Stubbs. "A Little Too Much of the Buchenwald Touch? Military Radiation Research at the University of Cincinnati, 1960–1972." *Accountability in Research: Policies & Quality Assurance.* January 1998. Vol. 6: 63.

The Experience of the American Friends Service Committee in Civilian Public Service. American Friends Service Committee, booklet 1945. Provided by Marshall Sutton.

Experiments and Research with Humans: Values in Conflict. Washington, DC: The National Academy of Sciences, 1975.

"The Fat of the Land." *Time.* January 13, 1961: 48–52.

Flynn, George Q. *Lewis B. Hershey, Mr. Selective Service.* Chapel Hill: University of North Carolina Press, 1985.

Foster, Claire. *The Ethics of Medical Research on Humans.* Cambridge: Cambridge University Press, 2001.

Frazer, Heather, and John O'Sullivan. *"We Have Just Begun to Not Fight": An Oral History of Conscientious Objectors in Civilian Public Service in World War II.* New York: Twayne Publishers, 1996.

Gandhi, Mohandas K. *An Autobiography: The Story of My Experiments with Truth.* Boston: Beacon Press, 1957.

Garner, David M. "The Effects of Starvation on Behavior." *Healthy Weight Journal.* September/October 1998, Vol. 12, Issue 5: 68.

Garner, David M., and Paul E. Garfinkle, ed. *Handbook of Treatment for Eating Disorders,* Second Edition. New York: The Guilford Press, 1997.

Garner, Jasper H. B. "Jay." "India and After." Published for the 60th Anniversary of his class from the Woodstock School, 2000. Provided by Jasper Garner.

————. Letter to author, June 17, 2004.

"General Info on Major Walter Reed." www.wramc.amedd.army.mil/welcome/history.

Gingerich, Melvin. *Service for Peace: A History of Mennonite Civilian Public Service.* Akron, PA: The Mennonite Central Committee, 1949.

Glick, Lester. *Civilian Public Service in Retrospect: Eighty-six Men Recall Their Peace Witness in the C.P.S.* Unpublished 1997 study found at the Mennonite Historical Library, Goshen College, Goshen, IN.

————. *My Legacy: Recollections of Family, Work, and Service.* North Port, FL: Lester and Doris Glick, 2000. Read at the Mennonite Historical Library, Goshen College, Goshen, IN.

Sources

Gordon, Bruce, and Ernest Prentice. "Protection of Human Subjects in the United States: A Short History." *Journal of Public Health Management and Practice.* November 2000.

Gordon, Danielle. "The Verdict: No Harm, No Foul." *Bulletin of the Atomic Scientists.* January/February 1996. Vol. 52, Issue 1: 33.

Gordon, Mary. *Joan of Arc: A Penguin Life.* New York: Viking Penguin, 2000.

Guetzkow, Harold Steere, and Paul Hoover Bowman. *Men and Hunger: A Psychological Manual for Relief Workers.* Elgin, IL: Brethren Publishing House, 1946.

Guetzkow, Harold, and Joseph Valadez. *Simulated International Processes: Theories and Research in Global Modeling.* Beverly Hills, CA: Sage Publications, 1981.

Hayes, Joanne Lamb. *Grandma's Wartime Kitchen: World War II and the Way We Cooked.* New York: St. Martin's Press, 2000.

He Served His Country During the War. Washington, DC: The National Service Board for Religious Objectors, 1945. Read at the Mennonite Historical Library, Goshen College, Goshen, IN.

Hinkle, Roscoe C. "A Life Career in the Polarities of Dissent." *American Sociologist.* Fall 1999. Vol. 20, No. 3:81–96.

———. "The Moral Beliefs of Brethren Young Adults of 50 Years Ago." Unpublished. Provided to author by Dr. Roscoe Hinkle.

Hoffman, William. "Meet Monsieur Cholesterol." *University of Minnesota Update,* Winter 1979. Available on www.mbbnet.umn.edu.

Hornblum, Allen M. "They were cheap and available: Prisoners as research subjects in twentieth-century America." *BMJ: British Medical Journal.* November 29, 1997. Vol. 315, Issue 7120: 1437.

Horst, Samuel. *Mennonites in the Confederacy: A Study in Civil War Pacifism.* Scottdale, PA: Herald Press, 1967.

Humphrey, Hubert. Letter to Committee on Character and Fitness. April 9, 1946. Minnesota Historical Society.

Jones, James H. *Bad Blood: The Tuskegee Syphilis Experiment.* New York: Free Press, 1981.

"Just Testing." *Health.* November/December 1993. Vol. 7, Issue 7: 87.

Kampelman, Max M. Speech given to War Resisters League, May 27, 1944, New York City. Text at Minnesota Historical Society,

———. "My Application for Minnesota Nutrition Project." Memo to Dave Swift and Adrian Gory, September 28, 1944. Minnesota Historical Society.

———. Speech delivered to Cosmopolitan Club at University of Minnesota as part of program "COs and World War II." Speech delivered March 3, 1945. Text at Minnesota Historical Society.

———. Letter to Elias Lieberman, April 2, 1945. Minnesota Historical Society.

———. Letter to the Honorable Birdie Armstrong, May 21, 1946. Minnesota Historical Society.

———. *The Communist Party vs. The C.I.O: A Study in Power Politics.* New York: Frederick A. Praeger, 1957.

————. *Entering New Worlds: The Memoirs of a Private Man in Public Life.* New York: HarperCollins, 1991.

Keim, Albert N. *The CPS Story: An Illustrated History of Civilian Public Service.* Intercourse, PA: Good Books, 1990.

"Keys' Army Ration Success, Blood Test Results Reveal," *Minnesota Daily.* August 8, 1941. University of Minnesota Archives.

Keys, Ancel B. "The Weight-Length Relation in Fishes." *The Proceedings of the National Academy of Sciences,* December 1928. Vol. 14, No. 12: 922–25. University of Minnesota Archives.

————. Letter to Frank McCormick, University of Minnesota Athletic Director, December 7, 1945. University of Minnesota Archives.

————. Letter to the Committee on Character and Fitness, December 17, 1945. Minnesota Historical Society.

————. *Coronary Heart Disease in Seven Countries:* New York: The American Heart Association, 1970.

————. *Adventures of a Medical Scientist: Sixty Years of Research in Thirteen Countries.* Minneapolis: Ancel Keys, 1999. Copy provided to author by Dr. Keys.

Keys, Ancel, Josef Brozek, Austin Henschel, Olaf Mickelsen, and Henry Longstreet Taylor. *Experimental Starvation in Man.* Minneapolis: University of Minnesota Press, 1945. Provided to author by Carlyle Frederick.

————. *The Biology of Human Starvation.* 2 vols. Minneapolis: University of Minnesota Press, 1950.

Keys, Ancel, and H. L. Friedel. "Size and Stroke of the Heart in Young Men in Relation to Athletic Activity." *Science,* November 11, 1938. Vol. 88, No. 2289: 456–58. University of Minnesota Archives.

Keys, Ancel, Austin F. Henschel, Olaf Mickelsen, and Josef F. Brozek. "The Performance of Normal Young Men on Controlled Thiamine Intakes." *Journal of Nutrition.* October 1943. Vol. 26, No. 4.

Keys, Ancel, Austin F. Henschel, Olaf Mickelson, Josef M. Brozek, and J. H. Crawford. "Physiological and Biochemical Functions in Normal Young Men on a Diet Restricted in Riboflavin." *Journal of Nutrition.* February 1944. Vol. 27, No. 2. University of Minnesota Archives.

Keys, Ancel, Austin Henschel, Henry Longstreet Taylor, Olaf Mickelsen, and Josef Brozek. "Absence of Rapid Deterioration in Men Doing Hard Physical Work on a Restricted Intake of Vitamins of the B Complex." *Journal of Nutrition.* June 1944. Vol. 27, No. 6. University of Minnesota Archives.

Keys, Ancel, and Margaret Keys. *Eat Well and Stay Well.* Garden City, NY: Doubleday, 1959.

Keys, Margaret, and Ancel Keys. *The Benevolent Bean.* New York: The Noonday Press, 1967.

Koehler, Franz A. *Special Rations for the Armed Forces, 1946–53.* Washington, DC: Office of the Quartermaster General, 1958. Obtained from website of the Quartermaster Foundation, www.qmfound.com.

Kromhout, Daan. "Findings and History of the Seven Countries Study." Speech given to the First International Keys Symposium on Nutrition and Health, Minneapolis Hilton Hotel, Minneapolis, MN. September 12, 2004.

Lacey, Paul A. *Growing into Goodness: Essays on Quaker Education.* Wallingford, PA: Pendle Hill Publications, 1998.

Laqueur, Walter, ed. *The Holocaust Encyclopedia.* New Haven: Yale University Press, 2001.

Lederer, Susan E. *Subjected to Science: Human Experimentation in America Before the Second World War.* Baltimore: The Johns Hopkins University Press, 1995.

Legg, Sam. Sonnet. 1945. Provided by Marshall Sutton.

———. Letter to Bob Willoughby, May 1, 1995. Minnesota Historical Society.

Leopold, Nathan F. Jr. *Life Plus 99 Years.* Garden City, New Jersey: Doubleday, 1958.

Lingeman, Richard R. *Don't You Know There's a War On? The American Home Front, 1941–1945.* New York: G. P. Putnam's Sons, 1970.

Lopez, Luciana. "Maryland Activists Prepare to Rally for Peace, Counter-Rally for Patriotism." Capital News Service. January 17, 2003.

"Major Walter Reed, Medical Corps, U.S. Army." Walter Reed Army Medical Center, www.wramc.amedd.army.mil/welcome/history.

Marrus, Michael R. *Unwanted: European Refugees in the Twentieth Century.* New York: Oxford University Press, 1985.

McNeil, Paul M. *The Ethics and Politics of Human Experimentation.* Cambridge: Cambridge University Press, 1993.

Medow, Norman B. "Discovery of Vitamin Deficiency Began with Milk, Limes." *Ophthalmology Times.* November 15, 2000. Vol. 25, Issue 22: 12.

Merton, Thomas. *The Seven Storey Mountain.* New York: Harcourt, Brace and Company, 1948.

"Men Starve in Minnesota." *Life.* July 30, 1945. Vol. 19, No. 5: 43–46.

Moreno, Jonathan D. "Goodbye to All That: The End of Moderate Protectionism in Human Subjects Research." *Hastings Center Report.* May/June 2001. Vol. 31, Issue 3: 9.

Mukherjee, P., M. M. El-Abbadi, J. L. Kasperzyk, M. K. Ranes, and T. N. Seyfried. "Dietary Restriction Reduces Angiogenesis and Growth in an Orthotopic Mouse Brain Tumor Model." *British Journal of Cancer.* 2002. Vol. 86: 1615–21.

Mukherjee, Rodranshu, ed. *The Penguin Gandhi Reader.* New Delhi: Penguin Books India, 1993.

National Center for Education Statistics. *2000 Digest of Education Statistics: NCES, 2001–034.*

"Notes on the Laboratory of Physiological Hygiene, University of Minnesota, Minneapolis, February 9, 1945." University of Minnesota Archives.

Obuszewski, Max. "Friends among 26 arrested trying to deliver peace letter to U.S. President Clinton." American Friends Service Committee, June 8, 1999. Available on www.quaker.org/peaceweb/kovdc1.html.

Pamphlet. Los Angeles: Committee to End Slave Labor in America. 1945. Read at the Mennonite Historical Library, Goshen College, Goshen, IN.

"Pangs of Conscience." Editorial in *Washington Post,* November 22, 1944.

Pappworth, M. H. *Human Guinea Pigs: Experimentation on Man.* Boston: Beacon Press, 1967.

Philbrick, Nathaniel. *In the Heart of the Sea: The Tragedy of the Whaleship Essex.* New York: Penguin Books, 2000.

Prabhu, R. K., and U. R. Rao, eds. *The Mind of Mahatma Gandhi.* Ahmedabad, India: Navajivan Publishing House, 1967.

"Prison Malaria: Convicts Expose Themselves to Disease So Doctors Can Study It." *Life.* June 4, 1945. Vol. 18, No. 23: 43–46.

"Rations: Conference Notes." Prepared by the Quartermaster School for the Quartermaster General, January 1949. Obtained on website of the Quartermaster Foundation, www.qmfound.com.

Research for Relief. Elgin, IL: The Brethren Service Committee, 1945. Pamphlet found in the Mennonite Historical Library, Goshen College, Goshen, IN.

Salisbury, Harrison E. *The 900 Days: The Siege of Leningrad.* New York: Harper & Row, 1969.

"Sample Form 47: Special Form for Conscientious Objectors." Read at the Mennonite Historical Library, Goshen College, Goshen, IN.

Scaer, David P. *The Sermon on the Mount: The Church's First Statement of the Gospel.* St. Louis: Concordia Publishing House, 2000. See especially chapter 14, "A Brief Treatise on Fasting."

Scholberg, Henry. *That's India: The Memoirs of an Old India Hand.* New Delhi: Bibliophile South Asia, 2002.

Scott, P. J. "Clinically Integrated Studies in Pathology: Their Contribution to Atherosclerosis Research." *Pediatric Pathology and Molecular Medicine.* Vol. 21: 239–57, 2002.

Sen, Amartya. *Poverty and Famines: An Essay on Entitlement and Deprivation.* New York: Oxford University Press: 1981.

Settel, Arthur. "Seven Nazis Were Hanged: The Diary of a Witness." *Commentary Magazine.* May 1960. Vol. 29, No. 5.

Shaper, A. G. "Reflections on the Seven Countries Study." *Lancet.* January 27, 1996. Vol. 347, issue 8996: 208.

Shaw, Teresa M. *The Burden of the Flesh: Fasting and Sexuality in Early Christianity.* Minneapolis, MN: Augsburg Fortress Publishers, 1998.

Shell, Ellen Ruppel. *The Hungry Gene: The Science of Fat and the Future of Thin.* New York: Atlantic Monthly Press, 2002.

Shull, Merlin C. "Ministry to Servicemen: A Classification, 1945." Survey data provided to author by Dr. Roscoe Hinkle.

Shuster, Evelyne. "The Nuremberg Code: Hippocratic ethics and human rights." *Lancet.* March 28, 1998. Vol. 351, Issue 9107: 974.

Smetanka, Mary Jane. "U Diet Pioneer follows his 50-year-old advice and turns 100 on Monday." *Minneapolis Star Tribune,* January 24, 2004.

Sorokin, Pitirim A. *Man and Society in Calamity: The Effects of War, Revolution, Famine, Pestilence upon Human Mind, Behavior, Social Organization and Cultural Life.* New York: E. P. Dutton and Company, 1942.

"Special Form for Conscientious Objector," DSS Form 47. Washington, DC:

Sources

The Department of Selective Service. Form read at the Mennonite Historical Library, Goshen College, Goshen, IN.

Starr, Douglass. "Revisiting a 1930s Scandal, AACR to Rename a Prize." *Science,* April 25, 2003. Vol. 300, Issue 5619: 573.

"Starved People Can't Be Taught Democracy," *MSJ,* September 26, 1945, 18.

"Statement of Purposes of the Jewish Peace Fellowship." Undated. Max Kampelman Collection, Minnesota Historical Society.

Sutton, Marshall. *Semi-Starvation Diary.* Written in laboratory, January 1, 1945–December 25, 1945. Provided to author by Marshall Sutton.

Sutton, Marshall O. "If Thine Enemy Hunger . . ." *Friends Journal.* July 15, 1985. 22.

Thomas, Norman. *The Conscientious Objector in America.* New York: B. W. Huebsch, 1923.

Tilles, Stanley, with Jeffrey Denhart. *By the Neck until Dead: The Gallows of Nuremberg.* Bedford, IN: JoNa Books, 1999.

Titova, Irina. "Leningrad Siege Survivor Recounts Detention at Camp." Associated Press, January 28, 2004.

Tuttle, Kenneth. "'U' Test Volunteer Describes 'Famine'" *MSJ,* 1946. Undated article in the Minnesota Historical Society.

Vandereycken, Walter, and Ron Van Deth. *From Fasting Saints to Anorexic Girls: The History of Self-Starvation.* New York: New York University Press, 1994.

Vanderpool, Harold Y., ed. *The Ethics of Research Involving Human Subjects: Facing the 21st Century.* Frederick, MD: University Publishing Group, 1996.

Vera, Rich. "Japanese War-Time Experiments Come to Light." *Lancet.* August 26, 1995. Vol. 346, Issue 8974: 566.

"War Stories: Lifting the Lid on the Siege of Leningrad." *Wellcome News.* Q1 2001. 26–27.

West, John B. *High Life: A History of High Altitude Physiology and Medicine.* New York: Oxford University Press for the American Physiological Society, 1998.

Wensyel, James W. "Home Front." *American History.* June 1995. Vol. 30, Issue 2: 44–67.

Whitaker, Robert. *The Mapmaker's Wife: A True Tale of Love, Murder, and Survival in the Amazon.* New York: Basic Books, 2004.

White, Paul Dudley. *My Life and Medicine.* Boston: Gambit, 1971.

"Who's Average?" *Healthy Weight Journal.* January/February 1998. Vol. 12, Issue 1: 3.

Williams, Peter, and David Wallace. *Unit 731: Japan's Secret Biological Warfare in World War II.* New York: Free Press, 1989.

York, Sgt. Alvin C. Diary. Made available on http://vol web.utk. edu/ Schools/ York/diary.html.

Zim, Herbert S. "What Happens When People Starve." *Liberty.* February 16, 1946. 16. Provided to author by Carlyle Frederick.

INTERVIEWS

William Anderson
Harold Blickenstaff
Scott Crow
Carlyle Frederick
Jasper Garner
Harold Guetzkow
Roscoe Hinkle
Max Kampelman
Ancel Keys
Henry Keys
Margaret Keys
Samuel Legg
Richard Mundy
Henry Scholberg
Charles Smith
Marshall Sutton
Robert Willoughby

INDEX

Index

ABOUT THE AUTHOR

———————◁○▷———————

TODD TUCKER attended the University of Notre Dame on a full scholarship, graduating with a degree in history in 1990. He then volunteered for the United States Navy's demanding nuclear power program, eventually making six patrols onboard a Trident submarine. In 1995 Tucker left the navy to return with his family to Indiana to pursue a career in writing. In addition to extensive magazine writing for such publications as *TWA Ambassador, The Rotarian, Inside Sports,* and *Historic Traveler,* he has published two books: *Notre Dame Game Day,* published by Diamond Communications in 2000, and *Notre Dame vs. The Klan,* published by Loyola Press in 2004.